How I Changed My Mind:

Eliminating PTSD, Depression, Anxiety, Fear and Other Issues with Psilocybin

By

Neil Holmes

Copyright © 2019 Neil Holmes

ISBN: 978-1-916820-23-4

All rights reserved, including the right to reproduce this book, or portions thereof in any form. No part of this text may be reproduced, transmitted, downloaded, decompiled, reverse engineered, or stored, in any form or introduced into any information storage and retrieval system, in any form or by any means, whether electronic or mechanical without the express written permission of the author.

Dedication

My dedication goes to those who have played an essential role in my life, having accepted me for the way I am and for being there at those critical moments in my life: Mum, Jayne, Nan, Jude, Pam, Malcolm, Riss, Paul, John B, Sylvia, Simon, Andreas, David, Daniela, Kirsten, Hugh, John G and Justine.

Thanks

I want to thank those who have been supportive and helpful while I have experimented with psilocybin and have guided me along the way. Above all, my wife, Riss, who has helped me on this experiment by talking me through complex issues I have discovered along the way, corrects the material and ideas I need to consider, making this book a little bit more interesting to read.

Also, for her patience and understanding, as I didn't give her much choice when I decided to carry out this experiment at home. I want to thank a good friend of mine, Hugh Ditmas, for reviewing the raw material, getting it into a readable format, helping me with my poor grammar and for the fantastic discussions we had considering different aspects of what I went through.

Special thanks go to my beta-readers, Nicky Bryson, Kiran Chahal, Dr John Goodyear and those who have requested to remain anonymous due to the subject. A word of thanks goes to my sister for helping me gather all the necessary family details from my past and answering my sometimes awkward questions about me and my past.

Another special thanks goes to Andrew Austin for reviewing my notes on NLP to ensure I have not made any mistakes or misrepresented this fascinating subject. And lastly, a big thanks go to all those who have personally experimented with psychedelics or scientifically researched the subject and have openly published their findings. Without you, most of this book wouldn't have been possible.

Disclaimer

This book details the author's personal experiences with and opinions on psychedelics and other subjects. The author is not a healthcare provider.

The author and publisher are providing this book and its contents on an 'as is' basis and make no representations or warranties of any kind concerning this book or its contents. The author and publisher disclaim all such representations and warranties, including, for example, warranties of merchantability and healthcare for a particular purpose. Also, the author and publisher do not represent or warrant that the information accessible via this book is accurate, complete or current.

The Food and Drug Administration or any other official organisation has not evaluated the statements made about products and services. They are not intended to diagnose, treat, cure, or prevent any condition or disease. Please consult with your physician or healthcare specialist regarding the suggestions and recommendations made in this book.

Except as explicitly stated in this book, neither the author nor the publisher, nor any authors, contributors, or other representatives will be liable for damages arising out of or in connection with the use of this book. This medium is a comprehensive limitation of liability that applies to all damages of any kind, including (without limitation) compensatory, direct, indirect or consequential damages; loss of data, income or profit; loss of or damage to property and claims of third parties.

This book is not intended as a substitute for consultation with a licensed healthcare practitioner, such as your physician. Before you begin any healthcare programme or change your lifestyle in any way, you should consult your physician or another licensed healthcare practitioner to ensure that you are in good health and that the examples contained in this book will not harm you.

This book provides content related to physical and/or mental health issues. As such, the use of this book implies your acceptance of this disclaimer.

Contents

Preface to the Second Edition 8

Introduction 10

    Apology 12

    Terminology 13

    My Opinions and Beliefs 13

    Who Am I? 13

    Before I Start 14

    My Life Journey's Key Battle 15

    A Breakthrough Session 16

    My Saviours 16

Day 01: First Experiences 19

    My Prescription High 20

    Mushroom Tea 23

Day 02: A Typical Micro-Dosing Cycle 25

    Dosing Patterns 26

Day 03: Micro-Dosing and Dark Thoughts 27

    Micro-Dosing Levels for Psilocybin 28

    Dark Thoughts 29

Day 04: Alcohol and Me 32

    Alcohol 34

Day 05: My Eating Problem 36

    What is a Drug? 37

    A Typical Day without Drugs (Internal Micro-Dosing) 39

    A Typical Day on Drugs (External Micro-Dosing) 40

Day 06: Light Dose and Its Effects 42
    Risk and Harm? 45
    Alcohol 47
    Tobacco 50
Day 07: No Dark Thoughts 53
    No Dark Thoughts 53
    Daily Scale 54
Day 08: A 'Bad' Experience and Toxicology I 56
    The 'Bad' Experience 57
    The LD50 Thing - Toxicity 60
Day 09: Ayelet Waldman 64
Day 10: Toxicology II 66
    Toxicology II 68
    What is a Possible Alternative? 72
Day 11: Psilocybin 74
    Psilocybin: Its Effect on Heart Rate and Blood Pressure 77
Day 12: MDMA 78
    MDMA 80
    Almost 'The End' 84
Day 14: No Contribution 86
Day 15: NLP 88
    My NLP Breakthrough Session 89
Day 16: PTSD II, Traumatic Abuse and the Psychedelic Legal Movement 90
    PTSD II 91

- The Difference Between PTSD and C-PTSD 91
- A Case in Point 96
- Day 17: Growing or Buying Mushrooms 98
  - Growing Mushrooms 99
  - The Difference Between Mushroom Types 100
  - Where to Buy Kits 100
- Day 18: Addiction 103
  - LSD, Alcohol and Addiction Treatment 104
  - Ricaute's Report and the Banning of MDMA 107
- Day 19: Serotonin 111
  - Serotonin 114
  - Serotonin's Negative Feedback System 116
  - Anti-Depressants and How They Work 117
  - How Psychedelics Affect the Brain 118
  - MDMA 118
- Day 20: Psychedelic Access and the Water Pipe 121
  - Access to Psychedelics 122
  - Death 123
  - The Water-Pipe and Cigarettes 126
- Day 21: Autism, Asperger's, Tourette's, Cancer and Chemotherapy 128
  - Autism: 129
  - Tourette's: 129
  - Asperger's: 130
  - Cancer and Chemotherapy 130

- Day 22: Yoga and NLP Breakthrough ... 136
  - NLP ... 137
- Day 23: Migraine, Ayahuasca and Religion I ... 139
  - Migraine and Headaches ... 139
  - What Is Ayahuasca? ... 142
  - Religion I ... 142
- Day 24: Who Should Micro-Dose and Why Ban Medical Testing? ... 145
  - For Whom Could Micro-Dosing Be Suitable? ... 147
- Day 25: Religion II ... 150
  - Religion II ... 151
- Day 26: Caffeine and cannabis ... 154
  - Caffeine ... 154
  - Cannabis ... 155
  - Cannabis Benefits ... 157
  - Potential Risks ... 159
  - The Legalisation of cannabis ... 162
- Day 27: Spirits and Their Physical Experiences ... 164
  - The Spirit Having a Physical Experience ... 166
- Day 28: LSD ... 168
  - LSD ... 169
  - Micro-Dosing With LSD ... 171
- Day 29: Lucy, Future Research and Illegality ... 174
  - Lucy ... 175
  - The Future ... 176

Day 30: Summary 178
    Summary 179
    Was Micro-Dosing Right for Me? 183
Sweet Spot No 1 - Guilt, Shame and Closure 186
    My Sweet Spot 186
    The Next Day 192
    One Month Later··· 193
Schizophrenia and Micro-Dosing 196
Sweet Spot No 2 - Detachment, Acceptance and Responsibility 200
    Six Days Later··· 205
    The Next morning 209
Possible Reasons to Legalise or Decriminalise Psychedelics .. 210
    Those Losing Out 213
    Making Comparisons 217
    A Possible Future··· 219
Sweet Spot No 3 - Self-Discovery 227
    Two Weeks Later··· 233
    One Month Later··· 234
    Two Months Later··· 234
    Eight Months After the First Micro-Dose··· 235
    Micro-Dosing Routine and Benefits 236
    Summary of Changes 236
    What Hasn't Changed? 239
    Other New and Wonderful Experiences 240

- Lucy 245
  - Psilocybin 246
  - Cannabis 246
  - How Lucy Started with cannabis 247
  - Cannabis and Psilocybin 248
  - Therapy Session 249
  - Alcohol 249
  - Smoking a Joint 250
  - Influenza 250
  - Reflection 251
- Sweet Spot No 4 – What Am I? 252
  - The Next Step 263
  - The Question 264
  - The Fourth Therapeutic Trip 266
  - Warning! 266
  - Let's Begin··· 267
  - What Do I Think Happened in This Sweet Spot Session? ... 275
  - Three Days Later··· 277
  - Seven Days Later··· 279
  - Three Weeks Later··· 285
  - One Month Later··· 287
  - One Month Later 288
  - Two Months Plus One Week Later··· 291
  - What's Next? 297
- Sweet Spot No 5 – The Master Reset 299

 Summary of Events 308

 One Week Later··· 308

 Two Weeks Later··· 309

 Three weeks later··· 310

 Four weeks later··· 311

 Five weeks later··· 312

 Six to Nine Weeks Later··· 313

 Eight to Twelve Weeks Later··· 314

The End 316

 Closure 319

Possible Uses and Benefits of Psychedelics 320

References and Further Reading 322

 Books and Weblinks 322

Preface to the Second Edition

For the second edition, I have corrected my mistakes and rewritten some sections to facilitate reading. Where necessary, I have included international weights to improve readability.

What I haven't done is, since I did this update just before the release of the follow-up book, How I Changed My Mind II, I haven't added in extra notes of what is to come, because this highlights how and what I was thinking and going through at the time.

When I reread this material after not looking at it for several years, it is pretty impressive to recognise how different I was with my issues back then compared to how I am today (after working through the next bout of topics that didn't arise in these sessions. This is another confirmation that it was the right thing to invest around 6+ years in dealing with my childhood past.

I now work as a psychologist in Bremen, helping those burdened enough by their past that it stops them from living their lives freely. It is my chance to give something back after what has been given to me, which has helped me get where I am today.

Naturally, life growth and journey issues are constantly changing, and we must be aware of a lifetime of growth through the highs and lows we all suffer. Not only that, once we have understood and learnt how to deal with what once bothered us, it gives us newer resources, qualities, and personality that help us enjoy those precious moments in life and find out how to pick ourselves up after we have hit another brick wall—this is a part of life.

This is about moving on with life with open eyes and minds, allowing us to form our opinions and goals that reflect our inner desires. Finally, we carry on once we find out what or who we are. The pots and pans need washing, we still need to take care of our mental and physical health, and we carry on with our everyday activities. We are nothing special; no one is. We are among many, and we choose what is right for us.

I don't know if I can say, "Please enjoy this book," but I can tell you to take from this book (and the sequel, if you have it), and use it for your needs and discard the rest. Listen to others, and decide what is ethically correct for you at this moment in your life.

Introduction

Each of us must decide for ourselves whether to put into our bodies what affects our minds, be it micrograms of a chemical, milligrams of a mushroom, ounces of an alcoholic beverage, or smoke from burning tobacco.

The Psychedelic Explorer's Guide, James Fadiman

Firstly, thank you for reading this book and sharing this part of my life journey with me, in which psilocybin has unexpectedly brought about considerable changes in my life and helped release me from a part of my burdensome childhood past.

Psilocybin has enabled me to obliterate my PTSD, depression, anxiety and other issues that have given me my life back. So, let me give you a brief explanation of how and why this book came to be, as well as the childhood traumas I have had to deal with.

This book evolved from a private project. While carrying out this 30-day micro-dosing experiment, I was searching for more information about psilocybin, and I accidentally discovered micro-dosing one evening while scrolling through the internet.

I wanted to know what psilocybin was and what it could do for some of us who suffer from various life issues that I was aware were holding me back. As I started to investigate deeper, I discovered more and more about other psychedelics, leading me to gain a better understanding of legal and illegal drugs.

In my younger years (during the 1980s and 1990s), I had only heard. I believed that the government position was that psychedelics were dangerous and that alcohol and smoking were safe for us, such that the independent information I was starting to find out completely conflicted with the government's position. This conflict of information led me to want to find out the truth for myself, not just concerning the risks of psychedelic trips and micro-dosing, but whether there could be any considerable potential mental and physical health benefits that psychedelics could offer us.

It was on Day 9 that I felt I had to restructure my micro-dosing tracking notes on what I had found out from another author who had completed a similar micro-dosing experiment with LSD. It included what other aspects to observe and what yardstick of comparison I should use from the first eight days of monitoring.

Restructuring my notes created inconsistencies and a dilemma that remained with me until the end of writing this book: how to present the information in a clear and understandable format. Should I use a standardised layout to rewrite the first eight days, or would it be better if the structure reflected the learning progression I had gone through?

In the end, I have decided to leave my findings from the first days as I have written them, as I believe this shows the reality of my experience and discoveries and gives the proper credit to those whose own experiences I have benefited from, which I hope will find some resonance with you.

Near the end of the book, you will find other experiments I have carried out. These experiments were to reach the psychedelic Sweet Spots, also known as the therapeutic/spiritual sessions, using optimal dosing with psilocybin. This maximum amount is taken without crossing that second threshold from therapeutic to heroic dosing.

The material presented here about psychedelics has focused on various respected authors' key findings from reputable and conflicting websites. I have also recommended various more helpful reading sources, should this subject be of interest, which can be found at the back of the book. In case you're interested in psychedelics but don't feel ready, I have tried to include some further options for you to review.

One of my problems was what to include in the book. The more I investigated this subject of psychedelics, the more I discovered and the more I could write. If I had written this material in more detail, this book would have become too big and bulky.

Instead, I want to credit the source and book authors where credit is due, and I hope this is clear throughout this book. With this in mind, please remember that this book is far from complete, and I recommend you carry out your investigation as you would typically do before putting any chemical or drug inside or on your body.

Apology

This book is quite fluidly structured, and I have waffled quite a lot by writing my findings daily as I have experienced them. I have described some simple activities that might seem tedious, but at the time, this had a substantial impact on me as I was learning about myself in terms of my abilities and limitations. In this edition of the book, I have deleted some of the more tedious sections to make this book easier to read.

Some sections may appear broken up, and I have sometimes repeated myself. In many cases, this is not just a matter of duplicating something, but considering differing views or taking the subject a little deeper.

So, please accept my apology if someone finds this book unstructured, boring or for anything important that I may have unintentionally left out.

Terminology
Throughout this book, I have been restrictive with terminology; for example, I have used cannabis to refer to all other names for this plant. This is also the case for the use of the word psychedelics. There are so many different alternative words to use, and I did not want to cause any risk of confusion.

My Opinions and Beliefs
Also, as you progress through this material, you may surely find that some of my beliefs do not fit in with yours, and that's fine. We should all take responsibility for our health and well-being. I think this also includes fitness, diet, and looking after our mental and physical health, without solely relying on someone simply wearing a white coat, whom we may see for a few minutes on the occasional visit.

I also believe that taking medication should be the last port of call and not the first option, as many of us tend to do even with minor conditions. I also understand that for some, there is no other option than to take medication, and have already decided what is right for us at the key moment in time.

Since I am not a doctor or specialist, I am not trying to influence you or anyone else. I think a certain limited number of drugs have a role in our lives, but should be used only in extreme circumstances, such as saving a life. If you have a different opinion or think I have been irresponsible in my comments or opinions, rest assured, I respect your views, too.

Who Am I?
Over the next 30 days and through the remainder of this book, you will learn more about me, my background and how micro-dosing with psilocybin has changed it for the better. For me to do this properly, I needed to dig deep inside myself to determine what had happened to me in my past. It is never easy to talk

about oneself, especially when one has overcome painful periods in life.

Until now, I have never openly talked about my past. But I hope that by opening up, some readers will be able to relate to some of my life experiences and the effect psilocybin has already had on me in defining a new way forward.

Until now, only those very closest to me know some of what I am about to describe as it appears in deepening layers throughout the book, so please be patient if it is apparent that I am struggling with this.

Before I Start

One thing I would like to say is that I know and appreciate that I have been fortunate for the life I have had in comparison to many who have been mistreated in far more horrendous ways than I had to endure.

Some unfortunates don't reach milestone birthdays, for example, and of those who do, many are left so mentally messed up from that abuse and trauma they suffered as a child that makes my childhood experiences seem like a walk in the park. My heart goes out to you.

What is important to remember is that we all have some baggage we carry from our past, no matter how large or small, and it is not our fault for what happened. What is our responsibility, however, is dealing with it.

I hope I speak here for all those children who have been inadvertently pushed over that inner mental threshold, changed us into something we should not have become. Also, my respect and admiration go out to all of you who fight daily against that unnecessary historical legacy forced upon them at such a young and impressionable age. I hope being open about my fight will help, at least, some of you battling through your life journey to free yourselves from the shackles of your past. This isn't the only way.

My Life Journey's Key Battle
The physical and verbal abuse that I suffered at the hands of my father for the first seven years of my life left me with permanent physical disabilities and life-hindering psychological scars. As a child, I had no choice but to absorb the violence, beatings, screaming, personal denouncements and witness even more intensive mental and physical abuse against my wonderful mother. This abuse pushed me over a key inner mental threshold that had a significant effect on my personality and my inner feelings of diminished self-worth.

As a child experiencing that violence, I learnt to accept it as a regular and everyday event that all families go through. The problem was that I had no other experiences to compare it with at the time. Before I was one year old, my father left me deaf in one ear and quite possibly with a leg disability that still prevails today. I've spoken with my mother several times regarding what could have caused this.

The damage manifested itself in the late 1960s, and the doctors called it a spasticity form of Pes Cavus (claw foot), probably not recognised at birth (we have a problem with this as I was checked correctly over at birth and all limbs were delicate), yet we still aren't exactly sure whether it's from my father's insessant verbal abuse that caused a neurological change within me, or whether it was caused by actual damage from my father's physical violence. The inner turmoil could have caused it, my mother was going through before I was born.

Maybe it was due to a combination of all of these that caused the disability. We don't know, even though we have suspicions. As a result of whatever happened, I had to wear an ugly and restrictive calliper on my leg as a small boy up into my early teens, which made me different from others, and I withdrew into my inner world even more.

As a result of being deaf in one ear, my other challenge was, and still is, that I can't determine where a sound is coming from. Depending on the background noise level, I find it challenging to listen to a conversation. These continual hindrances turned me into a confused, wild, and chaotic person, with bitter mental turmoil rumbling within the darkest recesses of my mind for the rest of my life.

That was until I started this life-changing experiment.

A Breakthrough Session
Later in the book, you will read a bit about the NLP Breakthrough session (Neuro Linguistic Programming) I went through several years ago, which helped me to deal with some of my past abuse. This session was an essential precursor to the changes I could achieve using psilocybin.

It was my NLP Breakthrough session that initially helped me to deal with the legacy left to me by my biological father, of almost fifty years of inner turmoil. The last time I saw him, as well as experiencing his wrath, was when my Mum finally and rightfully threw him out of the house when I was seven years old.

My Saviours
I want to add that in those troublesome years of mine, it was my mother who suffered at the hands of my father more than I did. Fortunately, my younger sister escaped his wrath because he was thrown out of the family home when she was still a small baby. Both my Mum and my sister have been my lifelong rocks. As messed up people typically do, I've mistreated them, ignored them and shouted at them from my befuddled inner world of thinking I didn't deserve their love and respect.

Yet, they have remained there for me to lean on when I needed them most, and words can't describe how grateful I am for their loyalty, support, trust, and love. I'm forever indebted to you.

So, I'll stop here and invite you to accompany me on my journey of discovery with psilocybin.

Neil Holmes
April 2019

The world is having a nervous breakdown. People are irritable, aggressive, tense, and anxious. Neurosis is on the march. It is galloping ahead at full speed, and no one seems to know what is going on and why. Above all, no one seems to know how to stop this inexorable march to destruction. Year after year, there is more illness, more suicide, more violence, more alcoholism and drug addiction. The world is coming apart at the seams. Valium is the glue holding it together.

The New Primal Scream, *Dr Arthur Janov*

Day 01: First Experiences

While the law of the land states that drugs are illegal to buy, to most of the hundreds of thousands of people who use them, taking medications does not herald a rite of passage, an act of wild abandon a surrender to peer pressure or a sign of broken innocence, it's another form of consumption, no less self-indulgent or meaningless than going to a restaurant, going to the cinema or shopping for clothes.

Narcomania, *Max Daly and Steve Sampson*

Finally, the Mexican magic mushrooms I have grown from a prepared substrate are ready. I openly purchased a grow kit on the internet from a European country where they are legal, and the company delivered the parcel by post to my home.

Although magic mushrooms and other psychedelics are illegal to possess and use in many countries worldwide, I also want to try to understand why international governments ban these drugs, and I want to find out for myself what their perceived dangers are.

These psychedelic drugs, which lie in the highest risk category in most Western countries, are supposed to be potentially lethal, to cause some of the worst unbreakable and robust addiction and to be of no medical benefit at all to humans.

Medical research on psychedelics has mostly been banned, too. But is this international governmental viewpoint correct? There appears to be a growing conflict between what governments are saying and the positively life-changing experiences that more and more ordinary people are communicating about their findings. Maybe the government doesn't want us to be free-thinking.

Hmm, there's a thought...

I am determined to find out for myself what would happen to my physical health and mental (in)stability by going down this psychedelic avenue with psilocybin. And the only way to find out is to test this psychedelic on me.

Another reason for wanting to try this experiment is that I have issues from my past that I don't know how to deal with, which still significantly impact my life, even at the age of fifty (as discussed in the Introduction).

On the internet, there are a lot of personal experiences documented (and several published research papers from the 1950s and 1960s) that indicate that psilocybin, amongst other psychedelics, used in micro- and therapeutic doses could help me deal with my PTSD, depression, weight issues, anxiety, low self-worth and some other issues I still have.

I also know that in taking psilocybin, I am going to have to go through a high, and according to the government, this is a significant risk to my health and sanity. But wait a minute, at some points in my life, I have been high on legal medication. What's the difference?

My Prescription High
I now know red wine (claret) is one of the forbidden five C's in avoiding a migraine, as well as the others being cigarettes (I don't smoke), cheese (I love the stuff), citrus (mainly used for seasoning) and chocolate (I love the stuff). One Saturday evening, just before the turn of the century, I thought having a few glasses of red wine while eating a delicious pizza with a good friend would be okay. How wrong I was.

I was in my early thirties and I had just completed my second week of a new job when, on that following Sunday afternoon, I was rushed into A&E with an intensely painful migraine. This migraine was triggered by the night before, when I had drunk a little too much red wine.

The pain increased as the day progressed, and I ended up rolling on the floor with such intense stabbing pains in my head that I was driven to hit it against anything hard (floor, wall, etc.) just to create some other pain-focused distraction.

It felt like the whole of my skull was trying to explode and implode at the same time. At the hospital, they gave me some powerful medication. I can no longer remember what it was, but it quickly dulled the pain that took me on a weird and wonderful kaleidoscopic trip. And I loved it!

At about two on Monday morning (I wasn't on a ward but had been sitting in an observation room for several hours), I was asked by a doctor how I felt. I replied that the pain had vanished and all I felt was a dull thud through my skull. I didn't tell him I was tripping, so they allowed me to go home, and that turned out somewhat problematic for me. When I left the hospital grounds, I didn't know how to get back home, and the simple thought of taking a taxi never even entered my spinning head.

At that time, my knowledge of the local area was limited to going to and from work, doing the food shopping and going for a beer. The hospital was in an area I hadn't visited before, nor had I paid attention to where it was in the county town. So, I started on my magical mystery tour home on foot.

I turned right, left, and right at random down the various streets. It was then that, as I misjudged stepping off the kerb while admiring the dancing stars above and around me, things started to go wrong. I missed the kerb with my next step, so my foot swung past me, and most of my body mass carried on going forward on its own accord. It was too late for my frazzled brain to guide my wildly swinging leg to stop me from falling over, so I (not-so-cleverly) tried to stop my 80kg bodyweight from hitting the road with the four fingertips of my right hand.

As you might expect, this didn't work as I had hoped. With my weight thrust on top of my fingers, I simultaneously forced each of the four digits backwards with a loud knuckle-popping sound I can still hear and feel today. I screamed my head off while writhing in agony on the road with four back-bent fingers.

Since I was still high, I thought I was confident enough to sort this little problem out quickly and effectively alone. I grabbed the four unmoving and throbbing fingers that were still bent backwards, pushed the palm against my thigh and popped them all back in at the same time in one swift movement. Boy, that hurt as much as the second scream I let out.

Afterwards, I decided to head back to the hospital to get them checked out, but I couldn't remember where I had come from. After a bit of aimless wandering around, I couldn't find the hospital and gave up. After several hours of further wandering, I eventually found my way home.

I didn't have time to go to bed, so I prepared myself to work with a sore and swollen hand along with an exhausted, thick head slowly returning to some normality. It was a long day in the office that Monday, I can tell you!

About a week later, I discovered the tub of spare tablets in my coat pocket, which the hospital had given me, in case I needed some more painkillers for the short term. What I wanted to do was to replicate that high again, so I swallowed the exact amount I had taken in the hospital. But all they did was give me a throbbing headache instead. I threw them away since they weren't giving me that incredible sensation again.

Mushroom Tea

So, I've harvested some of my mushrooms from the fresh Psilocybe Cubensis family and have finely chopped up 3 grams, equivalent to about 0.3g dried. To make a cup of mushroom tea, I've added them to some water to simmer for about twenty-five minutes. Numerous reports say some of the chemicals in the mushrooms can irritate the stomach and give a feeling of nausea, whereas drinking them as a tea helps to reduce the likelihood of this effect. However, unlike Chaga mushroom tea, I've also read that drinking the psilocybin tea has a disgusting taste.

Here I am, sitting on the sofa with a psilocybin or magic mushroom tea in my hand, and I am plucking up the courage to take my first sip, as I have had some growing doubts over the last few days on what could happen to me. Will I go psychotic? What about getting addicted? Will I steal and sell everything I can get my hands on to fund my potential psilocybin habit? Will I go crazy and end up a useless gibbering wreck?

I gulp down the not-so-bad-tasting tea while watching TV. Here is what I noticed as I continued watching the television. After about half an hour, the colours are a little more intense, and the sound is a little more precise, which is excellent. And that is it.

However, an hour later, I am still wide awake (near midnight) and feel fantastic. This euphoric feeling carries on until around three in the morning. I eventually fell into a sound and deep sleep. When I wake up a few hours later, I still feel great and realise that I haven't experienced such an early morning's energetic sensation for many years. My head is clear, my stomach is okay and settled, and my body feels relaxed. I mean, really relaxed. My new motivation leads me to tackle each of the tasks I have to do today with a more-than-usual level of enthusiasm.

When considering taking psilocybin, here is a basic summary of what is recommended for getting the most from them:
- It is easier to calculate the weights using dried and ground mushrooms than fresh ones.
- Dried mushrooms remain more potent than fresh ones, as more is converted to the psychedelic chemical called psilocyn when it is absorbed into the body.
- Dried mushrooms are less nauseous on the stomach than fresh ones (I disagree!).
- Most trippers don't sleep for the duration of the psychedelic experience. However, some think they do due to losing the concept of time and their immediate surroundings (aha, that's why I was still awake until the early hours).
- For a more intense experience, take them on an empty stomach (for me, it does not matter whether I eat or not).
- Eat something first for a less nauseous experience (for me, it doesn't make any difference).
- Around 2+ grams of dried mushrooms are needed to have a spiritual or therapeutic experience. This exact figure should be based on body weight and mushroom type due to varying amounts of psilocybin found in differing family types. See the first Sweet Spot therapeutic session for more information on this.

A micro-dose of 0.2g is my goal for tomorrow. Maybe I'll never experience this sensation again, so I want to make the most of today. According to the government, my addiction is already kicking in and I am at the start of ruining my life, mind and body.

Daily Scale: 0.5

Day 02: A Typical Micro-Dosing Cycle

It's a very salutary thing to realise that the rather dull Universe in which most of us spend most of our time is not the only Universe there is. I think it's healthy that people should have this experience.

Aldous Huxley

There are many government reports, anti-drug campaigns, sensationalised newspaper reports, etc, that say psilocybin (among other psychedelics like LSD, MDMA and cannabis) is highly dangerous and addictive, and more so than alcohol and tobacco. However, David Nutt in his brutally honest book, *Drugs Without The Hot Air*, mentions that psychedelics are one of the safest drugs to take. So, who is correct?

What I do know is that if I were in danger of getting addicted to anything, I would want to have it again and again once I've whetted my taste buds with it (like with chocolate, for example). So, this second day is an excellent early test to determine how much of a threat psilocybin is to me.

Contrary to yesterday's plan, I took nothing.

Internally, I'm still experiencing that pleasant, relaxed sensation from yesterday, and as the day progresses, I notice I am just as productive as yesterday. I am impressed by how it's still affecting me twenty-four hours later. Is there something in me yearning for more of these mushrooms? Nothing whatsoever. I feel good. And that's one of the reasons why I haven't taken anything. I like what I am experiencing and don't want to risk any change to it.

Dosing Patterns

So, how do other people micro-dose (more on Day 03, what constitutes a micro-dose)? In Jim Fadiman's book, *The Psychedelic Explorer's Guide,* he recommends following the pattern of micro-dosing on one day, then taking nothing on the second and third day. This first day off (the second day) is known as a 'transition day', and the third day is known as a 'normal day'.

Two reasons for these gaps help to track the effects of the psychedelics on us and to minimise any chance of becoming 'psilocybin-tolerant'. This dosing pattern is an excellent starting point for understanding Psilocybin's effects better before trying out other cyclic patterns.

Here is an example of a typical micro-dosing plan:

Week\Day	Mon	Tues	Wed	Thurs	Fri	Sat	Sun
Week 1	µD	Trans	Norm	µD	Trans	Norm	µD
Week 2	Trans	Norm	µD	Trans	Norm	µD	Trans
Week 3	Norm	µD	Trans	Norm	µD	Trans	Norm

Etc.

µD = micro-dose
Trans = transition day
Norm = normal day

What I like about this plan is that it allows each day of the week to be a micro-dose day, thus giving a fuller personal understanding of its benefits on performance, creativity, etc. Today, I implemented this routine for the remaining 30 Days.

Daily Scale: 1-

Day 03: Micro-Dosing and Dark Thoughts

If you want to go out dancing all night, stimulants will keep you awake. If you are suffering from physical and emotional pain, you take a painkiller like heroin, and if you want to go on an adventure in your head, you take hallucinogens.

Narcomania, *Max Daly and Steve Sampson*

Like yesterday, I have not taken a microdose today. Today, the third day, is a 'normal day' within the 3-day cycle plan. The body has time to recover from the microdose; in some cases, micro-dosers find this day to be the best of all three.

This morning, I woke up fine. Some of my night-time Dark Thoughts, those regular soul-dragging and life-restricting nightmares, have been chipped away or softened a little. I am still slightly more motivated today than my usual half-hearted attempt at life.

While carrying out this experiment, I am editing another manuscript for a fictional story I am preparing to publish. It's one of the best editing days I have had for a long time. I'm not a fan of this activity, so this must say something about the effect psilocybin is having on me.

I know it's early days, but if I consider how I am compared to before I started this experiment just a couple of days ago, I notice a slight improvement in my attitude. It's not much, but perceptible.

After a page or so of editing, I take regular breaks, five to twenty-five minutes each. Then, I attempt to edit another page, but the corrections get less accurate over time as my enthusiasm wanes. In the end, I have a corrected manuscript that still needs significant revisions, so the correction cycle repeats more often and is longer than necessary. This is not helpful.

Micro-Dosing Levels for Psilocybin

After investigating yesterday's micro-dosing cycles, I will explore the potential effects and impacts of psilocybin based on the different amounts we consume. The following weights refer to the standard types of dried mushrooms:

Micro-dose: 0.2-0.5g: Later in the programme, I discovered that my ideal level is about 0.11g. This amount touches the threshold that allows me to function normally.

Light dose: 0.5 – 1g: This range is generally used to help people relax and for those who want to enjoy more intimacy with their partner, for example.

Normal dose: 1 – 2g: This quantity provides a more intense experience without potential risks or 'bad' experiences.

Strong (spiritual/therapeutic) dose: 2 – 5g: For this dosage, it is recommended that you have an experienced sitter nearby.

Heroic dose: 5g+: This amount is not recommended for those who are new to psychedelics and is beyond the scope of this book.

Two points I recommend which should help find out what an ideal micro-dose is:
1. Buy some scales that measure 10mg (0.01g) or 1mg (0.001g). Jewellery scales are pretty cheap nowadays and are worth searching for on the internet. Dried mushrooms weigh next to nothing once the water content (90% is water) has been removed. And believe me, it's hard weighing a consistent amount visually or with regular kitchen scales, especially where there is a

high risk of accidentally stepping over into the heroic threshold.

2. To find the optimal micro-dose, I recommend starting with 0.10g (or less, if you wish) and increasing the dose in increments of 0.05g until you quickly notice within yourself when you have reached the right amount. For me, that's when I mentally touch that threshold. At this point, I feel a slight buzz in my head for a few minutes, and then this sensation disappears quickly.

If this sensation remains too long, I don't function too well, and I know I have overstepped the threshold too much. Then I wait until the sensation wears off, usually less than an hour, depending on the amount taken. Then I can get on with my day again with enthusiasm. Paying attention to your body signals makes it possible to learn the 'sufficient' amount quickly.

Dark Thoughts

One problem I have is regular soul-destroying, nightmarish Dark Thoughts that often harass me through the night and have a debilitating knock-on effect on the following day. I've had these Dark Thoughts for most of my life. Fortunately, these eased up a little after my NLP Breakthrough session (2016). Unfortunately, however, I was later to suffer a near-death experience that gave rise to a new type of Dark Thought.

In March 2017, I was rushed to the hospital suffering from acute appendicitis. My appendix was dangerously swollen, and it was ready to tear open at any moment. The operation to remove the appendix is a standard procedure these days, and was a success. My problem was that before I went to the hospital, I had unknowingly been suffering for a few days from blood poisoning (sepsis), and my body was in its first stages of preparing to shut down.

A bowel infection caused the sepsis and was extreme enough to warrant having to take a double dose of liquid antibiotics twice a day for more than five consecutive days.

This stuff is something I have avoided taking for my whole life because of the permanent and long-term damage it can do to our gut bacteria. Two different types of antibiotics were drip-fed into my body twice a day, and boy, it messed me up both mentally and physically.

The doctor said that it is standard to take these for three days as a precaution in the case of someone suffering from acute appendicitis and has had their appendix removed. If there are signs of sepsis, they should be hospitalised for five days or more, depending on the severity of the infection. Although this stuff messed me up mentally and physically, it saved my life.

Three weeks later, I turned fifty and was unbelievably grateful to be still alive (I still am) and having suffered no adverse side effects from the sepsis or the antibiotics. However, the antibiotics took nearly a year to leave my system altogether.

For the past years, I had dreaded turning fifty years old. However, after that experience of surviving blood poisoning, I was thrilled to hit that half a century. The only thing I didn't get to do because I needed to recover was to celebrate it with a party. I now look forward to each of my birthdays much more than before.

That experience made me realise how mortal I am and scares me silly. I still have not come to terms with my dread of imminent death in the future, and those feelings still haunt and penetrate my deepest thoughts every day.

Yet, what I had gone through hadn't dampened my Dark Thoughts. What are they, and how do I experience them? Typically, I dream of death, decapitation, disability, loss of life, stroke, heart attack, and more. It makes going to bed hard, knowing I have to go through those horrific Dark Thoughts prophesies each night, as I can't and don't know how to stop them.

As a result of micro-dosing, I hope to dampen these Dark Thoughts. Ideally, it would be lovely if I could dream of something harmless and more normal for at least a couple of nights in the week. Well, practically anything is better than what I go through each night.

Days Scale: 1-

Day 04: Alcohol and Me

It opened my eyes. We only use one-tenth of our brain. Just think of what we could accomplish if we could only tap that hidden part! It would mean a whole new world if the politicians would take LSD. There wouldn't be any more war, or poverty, or famine.

Paul McCartney

I measure out 0.2g of dried mushrooms for my micro-dose. I decide to take the lower amount (0.2 to 0.5g is the recognised range for micro-dosing). After my experiences with alcohol (see below), I think it is probably a better idea to be a little more cautious with the amount of psilocybin I plan to take and start with the recommended minimum.

I swallow the dried mushrooms directly from a spoon, chew on them a little, and then wash them down with water. Many say they don't like the taste and like to take them with chocolate, lemon juice, or honey, for example. I don't mind the distinct flavour of these mushrooms, so I decided to eat them without any extras.

After the first ten minutes or so, I notice nothing, so I start to edit my manuscript. After another five minutes, I notice the effect beginning to kick in. Suddenly, my brain gets a little dizzy, and my movements are uncoordinated. The best way for me to describe this sensation is that it is like that first light-headed sensation one gets when one has been drinking alcohol.

Even then, for me, the sensation is a little bit different from the effect of alcohol; the dizzying effect on the brain is milder, comes on slower, and is more pleasant. Wow, I guess I am now in a better mental state to work, think, and be more creative.

But I am wrong.

The amount is too much for me to correct my work. My eyes can't focus on my text, my thinking is scatty, and I can't concentrate on anything for more than a few seconds. Getting my thoughts into gear is impossible. My hands are jittery, like after drinking too much coffee or falling into a massive sugar crash, making typing and writing difficult. My handwriting is not legible at the best of times, and I struggle to read the notes I've written earlier today.

After giving up on my work, I decide it's best to lie down for a while and wait until this disruptive sensation disappears, or at least until it dies down enough for me to return to my desk. My stomach has a slight nausea effect, which doesn't bother me too much. Otherwise, I feel fine.

And how am I after an hour of rest? My mind is crystal clear, focused and relaxed. My hands are steady enough to type again, and my body is calm as I sit sensibly in my chair. The stepping-a-little-too-far-over-the-threshold effect has worn off, and I can now focus on my work with great clarity.

And what a productive afternoon I have.

If it had been alcohol that had pushed me over the first threshold as much as it did with psilocybin, I would have had more problems. I wouldn't have been able to function correctly for much of the day. I would probably have fallen asleep for a couple of hours, and after that, I would have felt groggy for the rest of the day.

So, in comparison, a weak dose of psychedelics gave me that dizzy sensation for a short while without the adverse effects of alcohol. I could work effectively once the effects had worn off, **and** I felt motivated **and** I was energised for the rest of the day.

What a turn-up for the books. I am already starting to like this positive effect psilocybin has on me in comparison to alcohol. Now I am looking forward to the rest of this experiment.

Alcohol

I'm as much use as a chocolate teapot when it comes to handling my alcoholic drink. In other words, I'm a cheap night out. I can't drink more than a couple of pints, I can rarely drink more than two glasses of white wine (red is a complete no-no), and I don't like shots or spirits as they mess me up too much.

If I do drink a spirit, then it's usually a brandy. But I take such a small amount that most people consider it a warm-up for their palate, whereas it's enough to get me drunk. The problem for me is that I become more of a prat than I usually am, and if I drink just a bit too much, I tend to see it again. This effect of alcohol has been the story of my life!

What I have learnt over the years is that once the room starts spinning, I need to stop drinking alcohol and begin drinking plenty of water straight away. I need to ensure that I continue to drink more water as soon as I start needing the loo in the middle of the night and again once I have woken up in the morning. Even then, I'm still at risk of a crippling migraine.

Sometimes, if I'm lucky, I'll suffer from nothing other than a throbbing head, and if I'm fortunate, it fades away as the day progresses. This is a rarity. Usually, though, it gets worse through the day and ends up being a right pounder by the evening. As I have aged, I have tended to select more what I drink, when and how much, which is not often and not a lot. It's a bit boring, I know, but I hate losing my weekends and the limited free time I have the following day after a hard night out.

There is more about alcohol I want to talk about, which makes me grateful I can't drink too much, but I will come back to that later.

Day's Scale: 1

Day 05: My Eating Problem

Research shows that people who abstain from using drugs do not make this choice because they are illegal, but because it is a lifestyle and health choice. Of those who do use drugs, the classification of a drug is of little relevance; apart from cannabis, two Class A drugs, ecstasy and cocaine, are the most commonly taken substances in Britain.

Narcomania, *Max Daly and Steve Sampson*

Today, I have taken no psilocybin since this is a transition day.

I woke up feeling reasonably good about myself this morning and prepared to meet the challenges I will face today. My work breaks are still too long, but the quality of my work is already a little better. I can put more energy into cycling and thoroughly enjoy the ride in the cold weather today.

Another thing is that my appetite has increased. Whether this hunger is one of the side effects of micro-dosing with psilocybin, as the munchies are synonymous with cannabis, I don't know at this time of taking notes. Another point I have decided to focus on is how it affects my weight and whether I can use psilocybin to reduce my addiction to crappy food.

I'm not fat, but I'm not thin either. I'm about 14kg (about 2.2St or 30.8lbs) overweight (OK, you could say that makes me fat, but not obese). I love good food. I love chocolate. I love creamy desserts. I love sweets and biscuits. That has been a big problem for me for most of my life.

When working in Hamburg several years ago, I reached a peak of 100kg (15,7St or 220lb), decided to act, and changed my diet completely. I managed to bring my weight down to a steady 84kg (13.2 or 185lb, but then over time, it crept back to 90kg.

My ideal weight is around 70kg, but I will be content if I can reach a stable 75kg by the end of the year, as this is the limit before I am at a higher risk of a heart attack. Huh, it appears the drug I'm addicted to is sugar.

What is a Drug?

The highly respected expert, David Nutt, wrote in his informative book, *'Drugs Without The Hot Air'*, defines a drug as a substance that is supplied from outside the body that crosses the blood/brain barrier, which in turn affects the neurotransmitters within the brain. He categorises drugs into four types:

1. Opioids, which include opium, heroin, methadone, buprenorphine and codeine. These are derived from the poppy plant and are mainly used as painkillers, as well as for those who have PTSD, for example.

2. Stimulants (also known as 'uppers') which include cocaine, amphetamines, methamphetamine, caffeine, steroids, khat, mephedrone and tobacco. These tend to overstimulate the nervous system, making everyday activities uncoordinated and more challenging.

3. Depressants (also known as 'downers'), which include alcohol, benzodiazepines and GHB. Of all of these, alcohol is the most common one in use. It's essential to understand what the word depressant means. What happens is that the brain 'goes to sleep', causing people to experience, for example, weak legs, slurring of words, poor focus and a lack of concentration.

4. Psychedelics, which include LSD, mushrooms, ayahuasca/DMT, peyote/mescaline and ibogaine. These substantially affect the serotonin receptors that

regulate our mood, anxiety, appetite, sleep/wake cycles and body temperature.

Ecstasy is different as it is a cross between a stimulant and a psychedelic. Ketamine acts like a relaxant and a psychedelic simultaneously. Cannabis works as a relaxant and as a psychedelic, too. I shall categorise these as a psychedelic in this book for ease of description.

Firstly, I include below the list he gives of the key communication chemicals:

Acetylcholine: regulates the sleep/wake cycle, alertness, and builds memory.

Cholecystokinin: tells us when to eat and is possibly involved in managing anxiety.

Dopamine: creates a feeling of motivation, drive, liking, attention, pleasure and enjoyment of food.

Endocannabinoids: regulate pain, appetite, coordination and learning.

Endorphins: create feelings of pleasure, reward and reduce pain.

GABA: turns the brain off and is involved in sleep, sedation, relaxation, anxiety reduction, and muscle tension.

Glutamate: turns the brain on; builds memory, regulates alertness, movement, sensation and mood.

Noradrenaline (Norepinephrine in the US): creates feelings of alertness, attention, concentration, raises blood pressure, lifts mood and can increase anxiety.

Serotonin: regulates mood and anxiety, appetite, sleep/wake cycles and body temperature.

Substance P regulates pain and stress responses.

A Typical Day without Drugs (Internal Micro-Dosing)

This comes from David Nutt's book on how we live with and without drugs, and I found it an eye-opener on how others think about this subject. Firstly, a day without drugs:

'... let's meet Ben, a clean-living man who doesn't like to take any drugs at all – not even coffee. As he wakes up and gets out of bed, glutamate is released, kickstarting his body's transition into being awake. He drives into work, getting stuck in traffic; it's essential he's on time today, and his brain is flooded with noradrenaline as he becomes angry and stressed at the thought of being late. When he gets to work, it turns out his boss is late as well, so he isn't in trouble after all, and a rise in serotonin levels makes him feel better.

As lunchtime approaches, there's a dip in his cholecystokinin which makes him feel hungry, so he goes to the canteen and his cholecystokinin level rises again. After lunch, he gives an important presentation, which his boss is really pleased with, and his being congratulated causes the release of the reward chemicals endorphins and dopamine.

On the way home, he has an argument with his wife, and his serotonin drops, making him feel miserable, but after going for a run, his endorphin levels go up, and he feels a lot happier. While making dinner to apologise, he cuts his finger and endocannabinoids and endorphins help numb the pain. As night falls, adenosine builds up in the brain, glutamate falls, and GABA levels rise, making him feel tired and ready for sleep.'

A Typical Day on Drugs (External Micro-Dosing)
And now, a day on drugs:

'...Jen. She does all the same things as Ben, except that she, like most people, regularly uses (legal) drugs to change her brain chemistry. As she gets out of bed, her glutamate levels naturally increase, but she also drinks a cup of coffee, which blocks the adenosine in her brain, making her more alert. When she's stressed about being stuck in traffic and her noradrenaline rises, she lights up a cigarette; the nicotine activates her acetylcholine receptors, calming her down. A glass of wine with lunch, (her cholecystokinin levels falling and rising again as she eats), elevates GABA, lowering her anxiety about presenting to an important client in the afternoon.

The presentation goes well, and she takes the rest of the afternoon off, supplementing the sense of well-being from dopamine and endorphins with the relaxing effects of two more glasses of wine. Her husband calls and they argue about whether or not she's safe to drive, which lowers her serotonin. Seeing sense, she runs home instead, stopping for a bar of chocolate, which adds to the natural endorphins released by exercise, improving her mood.

She's cooking her husband a nice dinner to apologise when she cuts her finger and doses herself with codeine to supplement her natural painkillers. Although it has been a long day, the adenosine and GABA in her brain aren't enough for her to switch off, and she lies awake for an hour before taking Valium and falling asleep.'

Once we start making these comparisons, it's interesting to note how often we micro-dose throughout the day with various internal and external substances. Several legal substances, however, appear to have more noticeably adverse effects on our health and well-being in comparison to those of illegal psychedelics. This realisation can lead one to ask what possible benefits these legal drugs, such as alcohol and tobacco, have on society. Surely, there would be many health benefits if they were legal, wouldn't they?

On that note, I think that's enough for today.

Daily Scale: 1+

Day 06: Light Dose and Its Effects

The more hysterical and exaggerated any Home Secretary was about the harms of cannabis, the less credibility they would have in the eyes of the teenagers binge-drinking themselves into comas every day.

David Nutt, *Drugs: Without The Hot Air*

Today is actually a typical day, but I misread the calendar, and it is now a micro-dosing day.

I aim to experiment and find out what psilocybin can do for me when I measure around 0.6g of (dried) mushrooms. When I experimented today, I didn't know this was considered a light dose (0.5g to 1g), even though I have already written in a previous chapter what they are. However, it was a good starting point for me to gain experience with what this magical stuff can do.

Some people recommend listening to music, meditating or asking oneself a specific and meaningful question before crossing the first threshold, regardless of the intensity level one aims to achieve. But music isn't what I want to listen to today.

I occasionally try to meditate, but I am not good at it. Sometimes, the meditative 'OM' helps me briefly, but that's it. On YouTube, there are various Om's to listen to, so I select a couple and set up my computer and headphones accordingly to provide me with around 2 hours' worth of potential meditation.

Out of interest, I want to learn more about myself and discover new aspects of my personality. I've learnt a lot about myself over the last couple of years since my NLP Breakthrough and want to build on my progress further. As I don't know what I am looking for, there isn't much more preparation I can do, so I decided to keep an open mind about what occurs.

I take my dose on an empty stomach, about eight in the morning and wash it down with water. Regardless of whether I eat something or not, it seems that mushrooms, or rather the psilocybin that gets converted to psilocin to cause the effects, take about fifteen minutes to kick in. This window gives me enough time to prepare myself: headphones on, Om on, eyes closed, and a blanket over me while I'm chillin' on the couch.

Firstly, I try to meditate by focusing on my inner self. That goes well and helps to remind me what I want to experience. I scan my body to check that I am physically and mentally relaxed. Yes, I'm ready. Then suddenly, I noticed a light sensation filling my head, similar to Day 1. And, suddenly, there is a wondrous flurry of yellows, greens, and whites; a kaleidoscope of colours that fits and harmonises with the chanting Om gently entering my only functioning ear.

The meditative 'Om' plays at 432Hz, and the beautiful and colourful integrated patterns whiz by. I forget about my meditation and enjoy the trip. After about thirty minutes, the first Om ends, and the second Om starts playing at 417 Hz. All the yellows turn to differing pastel colours of varying blues and purples as I fly through an oscillating tunnel.

I remember I am meant to meditate, but I find it hard to concentrate. Instead, I decide to enjoy this new kaleidoscopic experience. Being completely deaf in one ear makes it interesting for me that the changing patterns I see are happening on both sides (left and right) of my mind. I thought that being deaf on one side would distort the experience somewhat.

After about an hour, the colours and oscillations change to images, patterns and shapes. Most of these are lovely, indistinct forms. I'm still not sure, but I think snippets of my past fly around me, along with some not-so-beautiful images intertwined with the beautiful colours.

One image I have involves a cross between a wolf and an Alien (the creature from the film *Alien*). It is floating in front of me and is watching me. It doesn't disturb me, and I use this experience to ask whether there is something I still need to work through that is still unknowingly bothering me. This thing disappears for a short while, comes back, watches me for a couple of minutes, and then vanishes again.

At this point, I switch off the OM, and the silence allows me to explore my mind more deeply.

After perhaps forty or fifty minutes, I enter my body, as if I have entered my hollow self. I know how fat I am on the outside, but it's as if my inner self is encased in a hard shell. I ask myself what meaning there might be behind this. I enjoy the sensation of being inside myself, and it gives me the reassuring feeling of being more balanced. I stay within myself for about thirty to forty minutes.

The next stage takes me by a pleasant surprise. My whole body becomes a massive, sensitive sensory organ from top to toe. The slightest movement or touch against my skin sends fantastic shivers through me in all directions. It flows around, comes in waves and then settles down again before repeating itself over and over again. This sensation is one of the most amazing sensory experiences I've ever had!

After an hour of sensory overdrive, this incredible sensation leaves me, and I enter into a philosophical phase as I reflect on my experience. I don't find any real answers to my questions, so

I reflect on this remarkable experience for another hour. I enjoy this because I am not a person who typically probes so deeply into myself, and I find it interesting that I have discovered other layers to myself that I have not considered before. What I have seen in myself is a shy, quiet, and unsure person hiding under a false façade.

After this philosophical phase, I get up, have a cup of tea, and start to work with a level of energy and enthusiasm that I seldom have. I try to recall if I have ever experienced this before. My head is so clear. I am stable on my feet, have no post-mushroom wobbles, and my coordination is smooth and controlled. I am still sensitive to touch.

In summary, this is a fantastic experience that has exceeded all my expectations.

Risk and Harm?

Because psilocybin, in most countries, is in the highest risk category for drugs, along with heroin and cocaine, as being very dangerous, addictive and having no medical benefits whatsoever, I asked my wife if she felt at risk from me. She said no, I wasn't a threat. I was too contented and relaxed to be a problem for anyone, and she felt perfectly safe around me. I asked her if anything had disturbed her about my behaviour. Again, she repeats that nothing about me or my behaviour bothered her because I was so relaxed.

So, how dangerous are psychedelics in comparison to other drugs?

I have discovered two brilliant, yet simple graphs in David Nutt's riveting book, *Drugs Without The Hot Air*. The top chart shows us that heroin is given a rating of a hundred, as it has the worst mortality rate of all. LSD is assigned a zero as there are no reported drug-related deaths. Interestingly, magic mushrooms are given a one because although no one has died from eating edible psilocybin mushrooms.

The problem starts when an inexperienced picker harvests and eats the wrong type of fungus, which can be fatal. The danger of picking a poisonous one gives it a value of one.

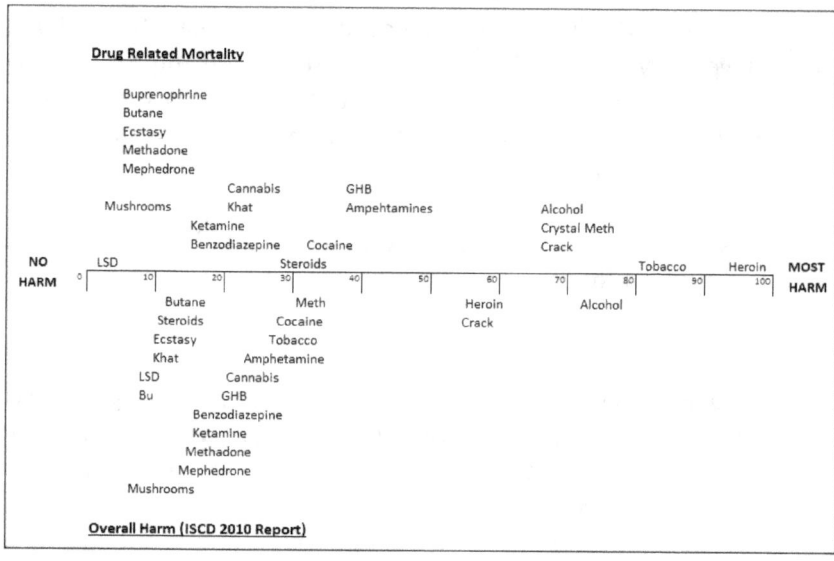

From the bottom half of the graph, we see that alcohol, heroin and crack are the most harmful, both for ourselves and their devastating effect on those closest to us. And again, when we consider the least damaging end of the scale, we see that two of the illegal psychedelics, LSD and mushrooms, are **the** two safest drugs out there.

When I first saw this graph, I was shocked to see how harmful alcohol and tobacco are in comparison to other drugs and actually how safe the four illegal drugs LSD, mushrooms, Ecstasy and cannabis are.

Within the remainder of this book, I would like to ask the reader to keep these comparisons in mind when considering the side effects and risks of other legal and illegal drugs available out there. For those who wish to take these subjects further, I have referenced my sources at the back of the book and have included extra suggested reading material for gaining a deeper understanding of psychedelics and other legal drugs mentioned in this book.

Alcohol

Let's look at both parts of the graph again. It may be surprising to see that alcohol is significantly more harmful than practically every other legal and illegal drug listed (except for tobacco and heroin). Yet alcohol is a licensed and accepted drug that can have severe and life-threatening effects on us. Nations worldwide, however, take these dire consequences like water off a duck's back. So, why is alcohol recognised and allowed, yet remains such a potential killer to the user?

In the UK (2007), we have around 40,000 alcohol-related deaths each year. In contrast, in the UK, there were approximately 200 deaths from all other psychedelics grouped, including cannabis, MDMA, LSD, Mushrooms, Ayahuasca, etc. About 350 people per year die directly from alcohol poisoning, and 8,000 people die per year from cirrhosis of the liver.

Another aspect to consider is the burden of admissions to the NHS. There are more than a million people who suffer from some alcohol illness or side effects that visit A&E each year. From these 40,000 alcohol-related deaths, there are about 13,000 that occur in individuals under 18 years of age.

Now let's widen the scope a little more. Around 7,000 people are killed in alcohol-related road traffic accidents each year. Around 500 include innocent passengers, pedestrians, cyclists, babies in prams, etc. About 1.2 million alcohol-related violent incidents are reported to the police each year, and this doesn't include the 500,000 or so other alcohol-related crimes, which cost the taxpayer (you and me) approximately £7 billion each year.

What about the unfortunate people who suffer the brunt of alcohol abuse that occurs behind closed doors? Around 40% of all domestic violence involves alcohol in some way. Sadly, approximately 50% of these are linked to child-protection cases. I know from my personal experience how hard it can be for a defenceless child to have to cope mentally and physically with a violent parent lashing out in an alcoholic rage. Again, this drug and its horrific side effects are accepted as the norm within our society.

This problem can be viewed from another perspective. In the UK, there are around 3.5 million adults categorised as alcoholics, with approximately 700,000 defenceless children in their care. These kids have no choice but to live with at least one parent who has a drinking problem. And then there are the mothers who drink while pregnant, who give birth to around 6,000 children each year suffering from foetal alcohol syndrome.

Another knock-on effect of alcohol in males predominantly between the ages of 15 and 24 years is that it encourages unsafe sex and the use of illicit drugs. It is also internationally known and generally accepted that alcohol is one of the biggest gateways to harder drugs and is linked to high levels of physical abuse and drink-related accidents. There is one more significant gateway to harder drugs than alcohol (no, it's not cannabis), and I'll come to that later.

Overall, this has a dramatic financial impact on the taxpayer. The cost to the taxpayer resulting from alcohol-related incidents alone is estimated to be around £30 to £50 billion per year. Consider how much less tax we would have to contribute to our government from our hard-earned monthly wage packet if we could bring this problem under some control.

Suppose we start to compare these effects and the costs of illegal psychedelics. In that case, the figures are a small number of 200 deaths per year, such that this could easily be merged into the government's NHS statistics without any significant impact on NHS costs.

Why? One reason is that it has been shown that when people take psychedelics, they tend to drink less alcohol, thus leading to less violence, fewer deaths, fewer hospitalisations, fewer pregnancies, fewer deformed and terminated babies and less family break-up. This saves even more taxpayers' money, which could be invested further into the UK's NHS system.

Fortunately, a proportion of the general public is now better informed, and many are starting to ask themselves why relatively safe psychedelics are banned, but relatively dangerous alcohol is not strictly regulated, with the only exception that you have to be 18 or over to buy and to drink it, however you like (in the UK).

What about the health benefits of alcohol that are brought to our attention mainly in newspapers or TV reports? We read or hear that red wine and beer are healthy for this and that, and spirits are good for something else. There may be a few benefits, but the other damaging effects significantly outweigh the promoted benefits when consumed in 'large' quantities.

Professor Angela Wood from Cambridge University says that a safe upper limit of drinking is a maximum of 100 grams per week (that's about seven alcohol units per week). This amount is significantly less than the government's recommended minimum. Some of the first symptoms regarding alcohol problems may include facial flushes, nausea, headaches and other uncomfortable sensations. In the long run, for those with a low tolerance, these issues tend to outweigh the short-term benefits of intoxication. I'm one of these people.

One of the most significant problems with alcohol consumption is that its key component is ethanol. Take a standard alcoholic drink, say, a glass of wine, beer, or some other spirit, etc. The ethanol in those drinks gets converted to acetaldehyde in the body. If this chemical were found at those same levels in any pre-prepared food product we would buy in a supermarket, it would be banned immediately for human consumption due to the health risks it could cause.

But, as I know, very few people have just one drink. The toxicity levels of acetaldehyde can rapidly reach critical levels. When acetaldehyde is not oxidised within the body, various illnesses can occur. Firstly, acetaldehyde can cause cancer. Some other problems it can cause are stroke, brain damage, cognitive decline, heart attack, heart failure, irregular heartbeat, hepatitis, fatty liver, cirrhosis, the risk of miscarriage in women, decreased fertility in men, pancreatic issues and wasting of limb muscles and even nerve death. Then there are the secondary social risks following excessive consumption, which can include loss of job, home, family and friends.

I'm not giving up my occasional glass of wine and beer, but it is undoubtedly a pause for thought on what we could inadvertently be doing to ourselves.

Tobacco

As with alcohol, when I first saw the graph on how much harm tobacco could cause a person, I was astonished. I know that marketing of smoking is forbidden on billboards in the UK to protect kids from starting up, unlike in Germany, and we are all aware of the damage smoking can cause from the pictures found on cigarette packages, which many have now grown numb to. Other than the requirement of being a certain age to buy and smoke them, it's pretty much unregulated.

So, what's in tobacco that could be causing so many deaths? To date, we know it contains more than sixty chemicals that are either toxic or suspected of causing cancer. These chemicals have been shown to cause different lung problems like chronic bronchitis, emphysema and asthma. And let's not forget to mention that smoking tobacco increases the risk of lung cancer by a factor of twenty.

Not only that, but the chemicals added to tobacco also constrict blood vessels, which can lead to heart problems, cardiovascular disease and a high risk of a stroke. The other knock-on effect is that smokers tend not to be as physically active as non-smokers, thus leading to a variety of weight-related and other health issues.

According to David Nutt, tobacco sales generate revenues of more than £10 billion per year. Health-related issues related to tobacco smoking cost the government nearly £14 billion per year. Again, it is the taxpayers who bear the brunt of this £4 billion deficit each year.

Then there is the damage secondary smoking can cause to partners, family, children, work colleagues, pets, etc. Around 11,000 secondary smoke inhalers tend to die in the UK and about 100,000 people worldwide each year. That's a lot of innocent deaths for doing nothing other than being in the proximity of a smoker.

So why isn't smoking treated as an issue like it is for psychedelics and other illegal drugs? One of the main reasons is that it is established in our culture and readily available for all to buy. Around a fifth of Britons smoke, even though nearly 75% of these smokers want to give it up. Almost 80% of those have tried at some point to give up smoking and have unfortunately failed.

However, we must remember that nicotine alone has health benefits, which are found in aubergine (eggplant) and tomatoes, for example. I don't intend to cover this here as it is beyond the book's scope.

You will read later why I don't smoke, although for a different reason than the ones given above. So, I wish you a good day, and we'll meet again tomorrow.

Day's Scale: 2

Day 07: No Dark Thoughts

I'm determined my children don't get hooked, which is why I want all drugs legalised... I say legalise drugs because I want to see less drug abuse, not more. And I say legalise drugs because I want to see the criminals put out of business.

Edward Ellison

Today is a transition day, so no micro-dose.

Through the night, I slept well and woke up with renewed energy flowing through me; this is an intensity I haven't experienced for a long time. I wonder if this is 'the new me' I'm beginning to discover. The clarity I'm experiencing in my daily thoughts is much better than before starting this micro-dosing experiment. Also, when I woke up this morning, I realised that I had no Dark Thoughts through the night. No nightmares!

Although nothing special happens today, I complete some good work and am happy with the results.

No Dark Thoughts

To wake up after a night of nightmares or 'Dark Thoughts' that consist of death, heart attacks, strokes, blindness, not being able to speak and suffering from partial to complete paralysis certainly makes a good start to the day rather tricky. But to wake up without them, like today, is a huge relief.

Generally, the morning following such nightmares, my heart feels like it is pounding out of my chest, and I can't breathe properly. I have a routine I follow each morning to determine whether I'm still alive and functioning properly. Before I get out of bed, I check my breathing to determine if both lungs are working. Then, I move all my joints to check if they operate.

If I'm not sure they are working correctly, I'll open my eyes to check if I can see and watch my limbs move. I'm completely deaf in one ear, so I check to hear sounds from outside with my remaining good ear, e.g., birds tweeting, cars driving by, people talking in the street, etc. I check whether my mouth moves and then say something. If it doesn't sound coherent, as can be the case first thing in the morning, I speak louder and more clearly to myself.

The order I carry these checks out each morning is related to the most intense thing I dreamt about. Finally, I test whether I can sit up on the edge of the bed and whether I feel the cold laminate floor on my feet. Once satisfied, I stand up to determine whether my balance is okay and then leave the bedroom, desperately needing the loo. To date, I've passed every test, but there will be a day when that won't happen, and that scares me.

This morning, however, there is a new lightness within my inner self and in my mind, yet I still do my checks out of habit. My heart rate is steady, and I am more relaxed than usual. I hear the birds tweeting and singing outside as I watch the sun rising in the east. A slight fear that I may not have checked everything quickly disappears as I stare outside the window, saying to myself, 'What a wonderful morning!'

After my much-needed morning cup of coffee, I crack on with the day's business, and again I achieve more than I had planned. At no time during the day do I have any niggling thoughts creeping into my head.

Daily Scale

You may have noticed that I have a Daily Scale at the end of each day, which measures my progress compared to before starting this experiment. I am rating my everyday experiences on a subjective scale of 0 to 10, where 0 represents my current level based on a typical day of mine, and 10 represents my imaginings of a perfect day. I give Day 0 a rating of 0 as my starting reference. Day 1 was an interesting experience, deserving perhaps a score of 0.5. Between Day 2 and Day 5, I have progressed to a score well over 1. On day 6, I would already rate it as 2. It's still modest, but it gives some hope for further improvement.

As a future focal point, I've decided to allocate a rating of 7 to the days that would match some of the best days of my life. This scaling allows for growth above and beyond my experience, should I manage to get that far. I must compare my experiences and progress with my personal history, not someone else's. Otherwise, I would rate the 'greenness of someone else's grass' with mine without knowing their whole history, which might be deceptive and a waste of my time. Not only that, my grass may not be green all over, but some areas have unique shades that are very important to me.

Daily Scale: 2

Day 08: A 'Bad' Experience and Toxicology I

Why should we leave it to organised crime to regulate these drugs?

Donald MacPherson

Today is a 'normal' day, and I have not taken a micro-dose.

I still feel good from my last significant psilocybin experience two days ago. I'm curious to know if this improved feeling carries me through the rest of the day as it did last time. Jim Fadiman, in his informative book, *The Psychedelic Explorer's Guide*, says that a significant dose of psilocybin can have a positive effect on a person for up to thirteen months.

That's just over a year of feeling better, happier, calmer and more motivated than before taking it! If this is the case, it seems to wipe the floor with most prescription medicines, which tend to have some effect for a couple of hours or a day until the next tablet is taken a short while later. And, according to several reports, there are no known longer-term adverse side effects with psilocybin.

Another way of looking at this is that if the 'side-effects' of psilocybin make me a more motivated and creative person for the next thirteen months following a single dose than in comparison to the short-term benefits of taking regular daily medication with all their known negative side-effects, I know which to go for. Which is better: to be illegally well or legally dead?

There is one negative side-effect to psychedelics, just as with legal and other illegal drugs, porn, thieving, etc, is that it can be mentally addictive. It appears that in most cases, any mental or physical addiction is linked to hiding from or getting some relief from something that happened in the past. Once this issue has been dealt with, in many cases, the craving goes away, and so does the habit. With Psychedelics, there is a slight risk of mental dependency rather than physical addiction, as with other legal and illegal drugs, etc. However, this appears to have a smaller chance of happening with psychedelics in comparison to different legal and other illicit drugs.

Surely, there must be some other long-term severe and adverse side effects from psilocybin if this is categorised as a Schedule I/A substance? Other than a possible mushroom allergy, there aren't any I can find documented. We take the psilocybin and have a fun, spiritual, therapeutic or good/'bad' psychedelic experience, or maybe learn something about ourselves over the next five to six hours or so.

It seems that the worst-case scenario is that a 'bad' experience can affect us, and we may panic, which puts us at risk. Afterwards, we get up and get on with our lives again, albeit differently. And for those with a 'bad' experience, it seems they tend not to touch them anymore for fear of repeated experience.

Admittedly, there can be short-term side effects from taking psilocybin (as with other psychedelics), depending on the size of the dosage. These can include dizziness, hallucinations, lasting perceptual changes, impaired conscious thinking, nausea, anxiety, fatigue, dilation of the pupils, altered perceptions of time, yawning and unusual thoughts. As I have mentioned several times in the book, proper preparation is the key to having a good experience.

The 'Bad' Experience

Firstly, let's define what we mean by a 'bad' experience. For most people, this would conjure up an image of something scary, reminding them perhaps of some horrific experiences that would be better to forget, maybe some phobia or a flashback from something disturbing if one isn't aware of them. We can if we encounter something that disturbs us enough to run away in real life. Yet, the problem is that when something occurs during a psychedelic experience, there is no chance of escaping it, which can cause some anxiety or discomfort for the unprepared. They might try to escape from those mental images, thus hurting themselves or someone nearby and ultimately ending up in the hospital, where nothing can be done except to wait in a quiet and sterile room until the effect wears off. Five to eight hours is a long time, depending on the psychedelic used, to be on an unwanted or unprepared trip.

Everything we experience mentally (see, hear, feel, smell and taste) in the session, regardless of how good or bad it is, we have experienced at some point in our past. The theory goes that our overall viewpoint on life, attitudes, etc, is also based on our inherited history from previous generations and what we have experienced. We may not, however, be able to consciously recall and react appropriately to these experiences once remembered, especially if we haven't managed to prepare ourselves properly beforehand.

The other potential problem is that when this terrible memory is in front of us, we need to be able to deal with it by learning from what happened. From my experience, having completed all my experiments and considering the experiences of others who have documented their findings, the most promising approach is to keep an open mind, as the answer sought usually lies on the other side of the problem in front of us. Only when we've processed the problem and internally learnt from it can we begin to understand and release those adverse effects that have plagued us in our lives.

Once we cross over the next key threshold (beyond therapy to heroic), then the risk of losing our sense of reality increases even more. Suppose we haven't prepared ourselves properly beforehand.

In that case, the risk of hurting ourselves or someone else, should we react to a 'bad' experience, also increases, and can lead to doing something stupid with a possibility of causing death. The risk of this happening with psilocybin and other psychedelics, however, pales into insignificance when compared to the effects of the many who suffer from alcohol-related injuries, for example.

In more cases than not, a therapeutic dosage goes more smoothly when prepared for and even when 'bad' experiences occur, we still have the chance of feeling different or having better knowledge about ourselves. We may not, however, want to have another psychedelic experience again, but that's a different matter.

Summarising, if you should decide to try out psychedelics at any trip level, it is essential to prepare yourself as much as you can beforehand. Ask yourself what problem you want to deal with, what solution you would love to have, and what you hope to gain from your session. It doesn't mean you will get it, but at least you may have a better focus and a stronger desire for change. Ideally, it is a good idea to have an experienced sitter nearby, as they should know what to say and do at the appropriate time.

For more information on preparation before a psychedelic trip, please read *'The Psychedelic Explorer's Guide'* by James Fadiman. This book is complete with information and examples on how to get the most out of it, whether for therapy, creativity, spirituality, etc.

For those who wish to be a sitter for a friend, this book provides invaluable information on how to be there when needed.

Remember, it's nearly 70% of psychedelic users who take them for self-therapeutic work.

But is there a risk of overdosing on psilocybin? How much would I need to take to die from this stuff? Let's investigate this a little deeper.

The LD50 Thing – Toxicity

Remember the saying some people like to use: ' A little of what you fancy does you good? ' That may be true, but how much of something is too much?

In the field of toxicology, the median lethal dose is written as LD50, where LD stands for Lethal Dose and the 50 represents that the amount (per kg body weight) of a substance, toxin, radiation or pathogen that could kill 50% of the people taking or being exposed to it, whatever 'it' is.

This LD50 rating includes all foodstuffs, preservatives, chemicals, drugs, and other substances we can ingest or come into contact with.

But how toxic is psilocybin for me, for example, in comparison to my wife, who is nearly half my weight?

For example, the LD50 is 280µg/kg bodyweight. For ease of calculation, I weigh 80kg. Thus, I would need to consume 80 x 280 = 22400µg (microgram) or 22.4mg (milligram) to stand a 50% chance of it killing me. A standard EU sugar cube weighs 5 grams, 5,000mg, or 5,000,000µg for a quick understanding of size and amount.

My wife weighs 55kg, so her LD50 toxicity level would be 55 x 280 = 15400µg (or 15.4mg). Still a significant amount, but as we see, it is significantly less for a smaller and lighter person. I won't go into the details on how the LD50 is determined. However, the internet is a great starting point for those who want to understand it further.

So, with this basic understanding, we can review some toxicity calculations of certain products to find out how comparatively dangerous psilocybin is (or not, as the case may be). Here are a few other substances with their LD50 value, and we can compare the toxicity differences:

Water: 90,000 mg/kg. Based on this calculation, I would need to drink 90,000mg x 80kg = 7,200,000mg (7,200g, or around 7.2 litres) of water for it to have a 50% chance of killing me. My wife, who weighs 55kg, would need to drink 4.9 litres of water for a 50% chance of it becoming fatally toxic. A child weighing 35kg, for example, would need to take in just over 3 litres of water to have a 50% chance of dying. Even water is toxic if consumed in large quantities.

Sucrose: 29,700mg/kg. The LD50 for me, at 80kg, is 2,376,000mg, or 2376 grams, or 2.376 kilograms. And for my wife, at 55kg, it is 1.6kg.

Fructose: 4000mg/kg: For my weight of 80kg, the LD50 is 320g, and for my wife, it is 220g.

Paracetamol: 1944mg/kg: For my weight of 80kg, the LD50 is 159g. For my wife, it is 109g. If each tablet contains, say, 500mg of paracetamol, then 218 tablets would represent her LD50, not that I'm planning anything.

Cannabidiol (Cannabis CBD extract): 980mg/kg: for my weight of 80kg, the LD50 is 78,4g, for my wife, 53,9g. Essentially, you would need to consume or smoke about half your body weight of cannabis in one very quick sitting for it to be fatal. Fortunately, it's a physical impossibility.

Death from over-consumption of THC and CBD is currently zero from statistics worldwide. A person typically takes around 8 to 10 µg per day of CBD for its benefits. To take a 50% lethal dose, I would have to be very, very rich to be able to purchase such an amount of 78,4g for my bodyweight.

Psilocybin (magic mushrooms): 280mg/kg: for my body weight of 80kg, the amount needed for it to have a 50% chance of killing me is 22,4g; for my wife, 15,4g. This amount doesn't sound a lot, but when you consider dosages are from 0.1g to 5g+ of dried mushroom that has an average content of, say, 0.5% (range from 0.23 to 0.90%), that's approximately 0.025g (25mg) of psilocybin per gram of dried mushroom. To reach the LD50 toxicity dosage, I would need to eat 8960g (about 9kg) of dried magic mushrooms. Our apartment isn't big enough to grow or store that many.

Aspirin: 200mg/kg: for my body weight of 80kg, the LD50 is 16g and for my wife, 11g. That's approximately (assuming 500mg tablets) 32 tablets for me and 22 tablets for my wife. That's not a lot of pills to put our lives at risk.

Fentanyl: 300µg/kg: Notice we have now gone from milligrams to micrograms, and the lethal dosage required is much less than the previous items. For my wife and me, the LD50 is 240ug and 165ug. One syringe can typically contain from 50µg to 1000µg of the substance. That means for my wife and me, the LD50 would be around one injection per day, depending on the dose.

That's not a lot, and this addictive stuff is given to kids, so if a child weighs 35kg, each injection could be lethal. The recommended dosage is 2-3µg/kg body weight for a one to three-year-old, but 1µg to 2µg/kg body weight for a three to twelve-year-old (reference at the back of the book).

I won't ask why the accepted dosage is higher for a smaller baby than a larger child. The side effects are the same for children and adults alike. Please don't research the side effects if you don't want to know what it could do to you or your child.

And lastly...

Botox: 1ng/kg: that's 1 nanogram! This amount is 0.000,000,001g per kg body weight, or if we go back to the 5g sugar cube: 5,000,000,000ng, we can better visualise how small this amount of Botox is. To reach this risk of 50% death, I would need to absorb... no, it's not worth calculating. It's a deadly neurotoxin; 1g is enough to kill more than 1 million people.

Enough said. I'm not going to use this stuff anyway. Although there are a few deaths and several more abreactions from Botox each year, I trust users have a good dealer who knows how to deliver it properly. Then there are other chemicals mixed in a Botox injection that may need to be considered too...

For those who are interested, for LSD, the LD50 is 16.5mg/kg. You can do the maths this time, but as you'll quickly see that the amount needed for a lethal dose is possible to reach (1,32g for me), it's costly to buy in such quantities. And if you did take this amount and survived, your trip may be something out-of-this-world, and if it turns out to be a 'bad' one, then the next several hours (or days) may seem like an eternity, and you may never want to do it again!

This LD50 system has a significant flaw that can affect us all. Although it is used worldwide as a standard indicator of toxicity for all substances on the market, it is also used to determine what is and isn't allowed in our medicines and food. But you must wait a few days before we consider this further.

Daily Scale: 2

Day 09: Ayelet Waldman

The War on Drugs was never about the drugs. If it were, there would be consistency and logic about which drugs are prohibited. Science and evidence would determine what gets banned. Instead, drugs have been selected for prohibition arbitrarily, and not according to which ones cause harm, or whether they cause harm at all.

The War on Drugs: A Failed Experiment, *Paula Mallea*

Dosage: 100mg micro-dose
Physical Sensations: Energetic
Mood: Positive, good
Conflict: None
Sleep: 7 hours, woke up once
Work: Productive!
Clarity of head: Clear and constructive
Dark Thoughts: None
Creativity: Very creative
Humour: On top form
Diet: stable at the wrong end of the scale
Daily Scale: 2++

Let me explain the reason for the different start to the day's tracking notes.

I have been continuously searching for new information on micro-dosing and from those who have had some psychedelic experience. I accidentally came across Ayelet Waldman's book, *A Really Good Day*, which I started reading yesterday and finished this morning. And I love it. It's written in a superb style, and I like her structured analysis, which has helped me to reorganise how I'm observing my experiences with psilocybin. Ayelet's experience is micro-dosing with LSD. I am curious to discover the similarities between the two substances and to compare the way LSD helped her and how psilocybin helps me.

So, back to Day 9.

I micro-dose at 100mg on an empty stomach today. The quantity is perfect, and I notice no nausea and no dizziness.

As a side note, a friend of mine, Lucy, started micro-dosing last week and found her ideal level to be around 140mg. Each time she takes a micro-dose, her energy level has increased, her work performance has improved, and she says her thinking ability and creativity have also improved. Lucy's problem is that she suffers from intense muscle pains in her neck and shoulders that can lead to crippling migraines, hence her interest in psychedelics. More on Lucy later.

A person I occasionally work with is my wife. One aspect we are working on is considering new marketing drives to reach more prospective clients for her business. Today, we came up with a new idea, planned it out, and had most of it in place before the end of the day. There are still a few odds and ends to sort out, and we hope to launch it properly over the next couple of days.

I mention this because during the next few days, I will mainly be involved in supporting her business project, and it will be relatively easy for me to reflect on the mental and physical changes I am experiencing.

Today has undoubtedly been one of the best working days we have had together in a long time. What would I be like in a year if this were the start of what I could achieve with micro-dosing?

Day 10: Toxicology II

I am convinced that the way forward for the human race is to recognise and protect the fundamental right of sovereignty over consciousness, to throw off the chains of our divisive religious heritage, to seek out forms of spirituality (or no spirituality at all if we so prefer) that are genuinely supportive of liberty and tolerance, to help the human spirit to grow rather than to wither, and to nurture our innate capacity for love and mutual respect. The old ways are broken and bankrupt, and new ways are struggling to be born. Each one of us, with our talents and by our own choices, has a part to play in that process.

Graham Hancock

Dosage: Transition day
Physical Sensations: Relaxed
Mood: More favourable than normal
Conflict: None
Sleep: Good. Woke up refreshed
Work: Productive
Clarity of head: Clear until I ate chocolate
Dark Thoughts: None
Creativity: I have sent off the manuscript for grammatical review
Humour: Light and funny
Diet: I am heavy and bloated after eating two chocolate bars
Daily Scale: 2++

Waking up this morning was a pleasure, and I have already crossed off a couple of activities from my to-do list before finishing my first cup of coffee. Productivity-wise, I have achieved more by the end of this morning than I had planned for the whole day. I tend to set modest targets given my limited motivation levels. This improvement has left me wondering whether I should consider increasing my daily to-do list. I have already sent my manuscript off for review this morning. This manuscript is the second part of a fictional trilogy about a country converted to mass obedience through the power of hypnosis and drugs.

I love utopian fiction, but this in-work manuscript and the first part of my trilogy, 'The Black Watch,' took about ten years to write. I haven't started planning the third and final part properly yet. The ideas are there, and I hope to get them drafted, written up, and released by the end of next year. If the effects of micro-dosing carry on like they are, then there's a chance…

One downer today is that I've scoffed a deliciously sweet almond bar with a cup of coffee in a lovely little café, followed by two mouth-watering milk chocolate bars with a cup of tea at home a little later.

One aspect that most relationships go through at some point is discussing one's differences, as I did with my wife. What it was about isn't important. We must nip it in the bud and put it behind us. Before my NLP Breakthrough, I used to argue a lot with pretty much anyone.

For me, nobody could be trusted, and all of them were my enemies in some way: my friends, family, partner, work colleagues, etc. In reality, I was my worst enemy and the one at fault. I would feed off the smallest thing, blow it up out of proportion, and then remain morose for a day or two.

In NLP, they say there is a positive intention behind each action, and my positive intention is that if I can keep people from coming near me and stop them from liking me too much, then I can't get hurt. Obvious, huh? It's a shame it took me nearly fifty years of my life to realise the futility of this way of thinking.

Toxicology II

Remember our discussion on the toxicology of various substances on Day 8?

Well, I'd like to take this discussion a little further. The examples quoted were based on standard LD50 values from an internationally accepted toxicological list designed to ensure that food, product and medicine producers don't provide us with anything too toxic that could kill us too quickly.

But there's one small problem.

Consider, for example, the product 'Adderall' (it's an amphetamine similar to the addictive drug Meth – remember the TV series *Breaking Bad*? Yes, that highly addictive and life-destroying stuff). It is used primarily as a children's medication, mainly in treating ADHD. It is sometimes used against depression as well as certain sleep disorders in adults. Its LD50 value is 15mg to 180mg/kg. That's rather a large window when it comes to determining fatal toxicity levels for our children.

Each tablet dosage ranges from 3mg to nearly 19mg of amphetamines, and it is usually recommended to take three tablets a day. So, if the highest dose is taken three times a day, it automatically could put you or your child over the LD50 value. Theoretically, it is possible to consume a few more daily before reaching the LD50 value, depending on physical build, size, constitution, etc. Nevertheless, fatalities still occur.

Apart from the risks of exceeding the LD50 value, we should also consider the effects when this drug is taken in combination with other prescription drugs or with certain chemicals found in some foodstuffs. In some of these cases, the chances of death, for example, can significantly increase. How 'significantly' depends on the other substance(s) taken with it and how much. For me, what is quite scary is that doctors willingly distribute this stuff to other people's children, knowing that it could kill them, just in the hope that it might calm that child's hyperactivity down, rather than finding out what the cause of the problem is. I also question how many parents are adequately informed about dangerous combinations with other drugs/food chemicals, so as not to increase the potentially higher risk of death to themselves or their children. I guess not many, if general practitioners are not advising us accordingly.

To summarise, the potential side-effects of Adderall in children and adults include: heart attack, stroke, high blood pressure, hypertension, arrhythmia, seizure, dyskinesia, exacerbation of Tourette's, worsening of tics, aggression, psychosis, mania and hallucinations, loss of memory, agitation, dizziness, headaches, fear, tremors, blurred vision, insomnia, dry mouth, diarrhoea, constipation, stomach pains, nausea and vomiting, hair loss, loss of appetite, weight loss, impotence, and death.

Who would want to put their child or themselves through the possibility of that when cannabis seems to have a similar calming effect against ADHD without the risk of paying the ultimate price? Isn't it easier to eliminate the cause of what causes such mental issues?

The estimated annual customer (patient) mortality rate per year in the US from Adderall among patients who have been diagnosed with ADHD is about 100,000+ deaths. It appears that some people have died from this drug despite taking quantities much lower than the LD50 value.

So, what could have gone wrong? Putting aside the fact that some of those deaths may be due to an adverse reaction resulting from a combination with other substances (legal or illegal, foodstuffs declared/not declared on food packages, etc), I will attempt to discuss one possible theory based on the way LD50 is calculated.

The LD50 value, which ranges from 15 to 180mg/kg, was determined by testing this substance on rats. This LD50 value is expected to kill 50% of rats. And only rats. Not humans. We don't know what the LD50 is for humans. If we do, I can't find it. As I said earlier, this value is used internationally to determine the toxicity of medications/processed food/other products intended to be given to you and me orally.

Still, I couldn't find anything about the toxicity of the chemicals we put on or in our bodies. This potential toxicity begs the question:

What about all the other LD50 products? Surely humans are not regularly exposed to the risk of death from drugs/foodstuffs based entirely on LD50 values tested on animals, are they?

Do you remember Aspirin?

This medicine has an LD50 value of 200mg/kg, which is equivalent to me taking about 32 tablets in a sitting. That's not many tablets that have the potential of killing us if we consider how many similarly sized sweets some of us can eat in one go. But still, the current death rate in the UK due to aspirin intake is around 3000 deaths per year. In most of these cases, the victims hadn't consumed enough tablets to reach anywhere near the LD50 rate.

Isn't that rather too many deaths for an over-the-counter medication? Apparently not. And this is without considering its other known side-effects: bleeding, abdominal pains, heartburn, headache, cramping, gastritis, ulcers, asthma, polyps, diabetes, liver/kidney disease, death and so on. And how many people have calculated their LD50 value?

None.

Let's take another example. Fentanyl is an opioid (also sold as synthetic cannabis – I'm still trying to get my head around this one, as cannabis works primarily on serotonin receptors in the brain) that works mainly on dopamine and norepinephrine receptors in the brain, thus making the risk of addiction much higher.

The LD50 value for Fentanyl is 300µg/kg. It has a history of about 52,000 deaths in the US alone in 2015. That increased to 63,600 in 2017, and this death count is expected to grow even further in 2018 (at the time of writing, there are no released figures).

Another example concerns chocolate. It is very toxic to dogs, but not to us. If dogs were used to determine the LD50 value for chocolate, it would be so small that the government would immediately ban chocolate for human consumption. I guess the same goes for other animals if they were used for toxicology tests with certain substances.

So, by selecting the appropriate animal, it seems possible to determine some level of risk to our lives that gives us a chance to play a certain degree of toxic lottery with our health. In other words, if a rat were ever to fall ill and a scientist wanted to save its life, they already know a heck of a lot about how to get it better again. With humans, however, it appears to be a different story.

The best example is to look at a toxicology LD50 table on the Internet and see which animals are used for testing. I've included a link to the version I used for the toxicology section at the back of this book.

A question comes to mind regarding kids with ADHD, wouldn't it surely be better to focus more on the child's symptoms and find out the cause? Couldn't the doctor (or rather shouldn't the doctor) first try to eliminate the potential cause(s) with the help of the parent(s) or guardian(s)? Maybe that would include removing all processed and sugary foods from their diet, eliminating unnecessary medication, changing lifestyle, etc.

Then, if there seems to be no benefit from doing that, perhaps prescribing cannabis or other psychedelics that have the potential to help without the risk of death and other potentially devastating side effects, before progressing to such medicine. Isn't this the reason we have doctors? Isn't prevention better than continuously implementing the 'cover-up cure'?

What is a Possible Alternative?

Another possible alternative to determining a drug's potential and risks is the calculated 'therapy ratio'. This therapy ratio figure helps to determine the amount of the drug that causes possible toxicity, as well as its success rate. Essentially, the larger the therapy ratio number, the safer the drug. For example, psilocybin has a high therapeutic ratio of 1:1000.

If we compare this with aspirin (1:199) and tobacco (1:21), we can instantly see the difference in assessing our risks when taking any drug. Fortunately, this is a relatively simple figure to calculate for a scientist or doctor. Unfortunately, for the average person, these values are controlled by a private company for some reason, and the complete values aren't available for us to review.

Hmm, what are they trying not to tell us about their products?

If we base our medicines on this value, it could help decide which medication is more appropriate for each customer (patient). As an example, cannabis is the highest of all drugs. This is between 1:10,000 and 1:40,000. Since no one has died from cannabis, as it is practically impossible to take an overdose, it is deemed very safe.

Let's investigate this more deeply to see how practical this ratio value is. Alcohol, for example, has a therapeutic ratio of 1:10. This value, simplistically speaking, means if it takes one shot to get you drunk, then you would need ten shots to kill you. This ratio helps to decide what is safer to take and what isn't. Back to psilocybin with a ratio of 1:1,000, we infer that if 10g is needed for me to go into an intense trance, then 10,000g or 10kg of mushrooms is required to kill me.

One of the reasons for psilocybin having an incredibly high ratio figure, but not as high as cannabis, is that this calculation is based on the deaths of inexperienced harvesters picking and eating poisonous psilocybin mushrooms. But why include other non-related mushroom deaths in this figure due to some uneducated mistake? It appears we don't do this with other drugs and substances, which is also a case of mistaken identity, so why here?

Here is another example to consider on the merits of aspirin versus cannabis. Cannabis is ten times more effective than aspirin. The therapeutic ratio of cannabis is 1:10,000-1:40,000, and aspirin is 1:199. Thus, the risk of death and other side effects from aspirin is much higher than for cannabis unless a 1-ton bale of cannabis happens to fall on you.

Aspirin is a processed drug with potentially fatal side effects. Yet, cannabis is a natural plant with more than a hundred different discrete cannabinoids that are currently known to support each other for our overall health.

What I like is the potential of its positive effect on the mind and body, especially having that personal comfort that it is possibly fighting against illnesses and cancers we may not know we have. When we make comparisons like this, it suddenly becomes a no-brainer, which is preferable. All we now need is for the government to verify it scientifically.

Day 11: Psilocybin

'I have been born again,' he told the astonished reporters. 'I have been through a psychiatric experience which has completely changed me. I was horrendous. I had to face things about myself which I never admitted, which I didn't know were there. Now I know that I hurt every woman I ever loved. I was an utter fake, a self-opinionated bore, a know-all who knew very little. 'I found I was hiding behind all kinds of defences, hypocrisies and vanities. I had to get rid of them layer by layer. The moment when your conscious meets your subconscious is a hell of a wrench. With me, there came a day when I saw the light'.

Cary Grant

Dosage: Normal day
Physical Sensations: Energetic
Mood: Good
Conflict: None
Sleep: Good
Work: Active and constructive
Clarity of head: Focused
Dark Thoughts: None
Creativity: Little, but being switched on to surrounding problems and proactively responding
Humour: Good
Diet: Started well, but ended up munching on chocolates through most of the day
Daily Scale: 2++

Upon waking up, the throbbing on the right side of my head is a sure reminder that I had exceeded my beer limit last night. This type of throbbing is usually a bad sign. My headache usually becomes a migraine and could progressively worsen throughout the day.

I came home last night in a light stupor and went straight to bed, forgetting to drink some water. Upon waking up, I staggered towards the kitchen in the morning to brew my much-needed coffee. Before I arrived, my wife asked me what I thought about new ideas for expanding the marketing strategy we developed yesterday. Quickly, we got into a discussion and started reviewing her latest ideas. This conversation flows and is productive.

After this exchange of ideas, it's coffee time. I usually don't function well without my coffee in the morning, but we both achieve a lot quickly. And as I make my coffee, I notice my head is starting to clear up. Being mentally switched on so quickly is a rarity for me.

So, coffee absorbed, and I am feeling more human again. Then I realise I must head into the city to gather information about my wife's marketing strategy. I had also promised a friend to help him in his restaurant at lunchtime, so time is tight. I jump into a tram and dash into the city since the weather is -5 °C outside, sort out what I need to do and head back home on the bus in good time.

We review the information I have gathered, and once we have made our decisions, I ring the organisers and say I will come by and show them our marketing plan and material around four in the afternoon.

After doing other jobs, I shower and head to my friend's restaurant by bike. It's still -5 °C, sunny, and the sky is blue; it's only a ten-minute ride from where we live, and I enjoy the short journey there. It's the first time I've helped him manage the till while he serves the customers because of a staffing shortage.

He's an excellent cook and likes to serve the food in a specific style. That's fine. I learn how to use the till and get on with the job. The place is packed with a continuous stream of lunchtime customers.

Ultimately, I do not just work the till but also serve customers food, stock up on cutlery, and do any other urgent odd jobs that need to be done.

The place quieted after a few hours, and we were sold out of everything. He says this is a first for him in a few months; he has been running his restaurant. I have helped him out before, and usually once the restaurant quietens, we drink a coffee together and chat, but today, I need to leave in good time. I head home, grab something quick to eat, and dash out into the cold again.

I jump on the bus and head into the city. It's warming up a little, now -4°C outside. I plan to meet up with a friend for a few drinks afterwards. Setting up my wife's marketing display is straightforward and quite therapeutic.

My wife has decided how she wants it laid out and has printed out the necessary display materials. After an hour or so, I finish setting up and am pleased with how it looks. It requires a few minor changes, but those will be done tomorrow when I have the remaining material I couldn't pick up today.

After that, I headed into town to meet a friend, and what a lovely evening it turned out to be.

Overall, I'm impressed with the day, and I have such a level of motivation I haven't had in a long time.

Psilocybin: Its Effect on Heart Rate and Blood Pressure

During our conversation, my friend asks me about the effect of psilocybin on the heart and blood pressure, which is a good question.

Firstly, I need to think about what happened to me. I notice no changes in my heart rate or blood pressure when micro-dosing. I have occasionally measured them before, during, and after a micro-dose, and they are consistently stable.

Once I step over the first threshold, I notice my heart rate increases its tempo slightly and pounds a little stronger for several beats before calming down again. Within less than a minute, my heart is functioning normally again, and there is no noticeable aggressiveness. One theory is that after the initial rush, psilocybin helps relax the blood vessels and allows the blood to flow through the body more easily. Because of this, it helps against migraines and headaches, too.

So, in summary, for individuals taking an over-the-threshold psilocybin dose, there appear to be no apparent ill effects on the heart. On the other hand, there seem to be many mental and physical health benefits. If someone suffers from high blood pressure, however, it may make sense to normalise this first before starting to micro-dose and speak to a doctor or someone qualified to help.

Day 12: MDMA

I think MDMA-assisted psychotherapy is one of the most important things we need to be focusing on in terms of mental health. It blows every other treatment for PTSD out of the water.

James Casey (Psychedelics Today)

Dosage: Micro-dose 100mg
Physical Sensations: Relaxed
Mood: OK
Conflict: None
Sleep: Short, but woke up fine on little sleep
Work: Busy and constructive
Clarity of head: Clear and functioning
Dark Thoughts: None
Creativity: Goods
Humour: Pleasant
Diet: Feel bloated
Daily Scale: 2++

My night is horrendous, and I can't sleep. My heart feels like it is pounding out of my chest, almost to the point of hurting. Talk about a sugar overdose from the day before (I ate a lot of chocolate from some (a lot of) sweets my friend brought me). At around one in the morning, I trundle into the living room and read a book until about three in the morning when my heart drops to a regular and softer rhythm, so I can finally go to bed to sleep. I don't expect to wake up fresh; my head is as clear as a bell. And I am up earlier than usual. 'I feel good,' to quote James Brown.

Today turns out to be another productive day, too. I plan to finish my wife's marketing display in the city with a more prominent poster than the temporary one she printed yesterday. My main job for today is to organise that poster at a printer's shop before visiting a friend. After sorting out a few odd jobs at home, I shoot into the city to the printer's shop I usually use. But for some unknown reason, it's closed.

The problem is I don't know where another printer's shop can be found. It's not a thing I need all that often. I pop into a local café with Wi-Fi and buy a coffee to search for one on my mobile. As my coffee arrived, I realised I had forgotten my mobile and had no internet access. I down the hot coffee and dash out to hunt for a telephone box to ring my wife to ask her to search for a printer's shop on her computer at home. But there are so few around nowadays that it took a while to find one.

With time running out, I find a printer's shop that offers complete printing services. I ask the guy behind the counter whether he does A2. He does, and I ask him if he can do one copy of two different print-outs for me. His reply is yes, in principle, but he has too much to do. Can I pick up the two copies on Monday? He has a mug of coffee in one hand and a sandwich in the other, and the shop is empty.

OK, it's Friday, and his enthusiasm is probably waiting for the weekend to start, but it's just gone one in the afternoon, and his shop doesn't close until five. I leave a little confused and irritated, but after wildly searching the streets in the area, I find another printer's shop willing to fulfil my request immediately.

They are so good that they have become our primary printer source for future work. Through their expertise, they could print the much-needed poster in A1 format instead of A2 without losing any detail, which is better for the overall aesthetics of the display.

Later, I joined my wife with the impressive prints at our pre-arranged time. After we updated the marketing display, we both agreed it looked stunning.

We head home in a good mood, feeling we have achieved something today. In my wife's office, we created some other incentive literature to be used in conjunction with the poster, and they turned out fantastically and looked much better than expected.

All in all, it has been a good day. The micro-dosing effect on me is fantastic. I am more buoyant, relaxed, energetic, and optimistic. My wife says she is feeding off my improved energy levels and helping her achieve more herself, too. I try to remember when I last felt like this. It was a long, long time ago.

The only thing that's not working according to plan is my eating. This diet needs some serious attention, but I'm unsure how to go about it.

MDMA

MDMA, or 'Molly', is also known as 'Ecstasy', and is primarily used as a recreational or party drug with the effects lasting between 3-6 hours. According to the government, as with other psychedelics, it has no formally accepted medical uses. But just as with other psychedelics, I find a lot of conflicting information about its potential benefits documented out there.

Let's also give it its other name, besides 'Adam', it is called the 'love drug'. It generates high levels of euphoria and increases feelings of empathy and closeness with others and oneself. It also helps with relaxation, reduces anxiety, induces a higher emotional response, gives mild hallucinations, enhances perceptions, and heightens sensations.

The first time I had heard about this drug was after the unfortunate death of Leah Betts in the mid-1990s, who had taken two Ecstasy tablets at the same time. At that time, the UK government wasn't providing enough information on how to deal with the potential risks of psychedelic use. They were more concerned about waging war against these powerful drugs than ensuring the safety of party-goers, where a percentage of them are going to take something, legal or otherwise. This girl naturally relied on the limited and mixed information from friends she had received to stay hydrated. Because she wasn't feeling too well, she drank about 7 litres (about 12 UK pints) of water in around 90 minutes.

Her LD50 value for water, based on her weight, which I guess was no more than 70kg (I think she weighed a bit less), was around six litres. The amount of water she drank, independent of the MDMA taken, is what killed the poor girl. This excess water affected her sodium by pushing it to seriously low levels.

It's hard to imagine, but all that water she had drunk was sucked up into her brain. Naturally, this absorption of water caused her brain to swell, which, in turn, put immense pressure on her brain stem, and unfortunately, she quickly fell into a coma from which she never recovered. My condolences go to her parents for the loss of their wonderful child.

Although too late for Leah and others, the government started to improve their public health campaign by recommending that Ecstasy users sip water at a rate of 1 UK pint (a little more than half a litre) an hour. The other bit of good advice is to keep a better sodium balance, too. Users should drink either an isotonic sports drink or water with added salt (rock or sea salt). This simple piece of advice has since helped to reduce the overall number of deaths from the use of Ecstasy.

Although it rarely occurs, MDMA-related deaths among users can be due to liver failure, kidney failure, heart failure, blood clots, brain haemorrhage, too little water (dehydration), too much water (hyponatremia) and allergic reactions. What I am not sure of is whether these points are linked to the MDMA itself or other ingredients it is mixed with to make the tablet.

Although it is a significant loss when anybody dies, the rate of deaths from MDMA is significantly less than those who die from over-the-counter aspirin. In the UK, there are at least three thousand aspirin deaths per year in comparison to eight MDMA deaths per year.

With this psychedelic, the one point I have come across is that there is a slight increase in the heart rate, especially for those who may have heart issues.

Some of us, however, may have difficulty understanding what a potentially dangerous drug is and what isn't, irrespective of whether it is legal or not, due to all the mixed messages flying around.

Politicians, on the other hand, don't like scientists making comparisons between legal and illegal drugs. Jacqui Smith, a British MP, once berated David Nutt, who was once a government advisor, by telling him, 'You can't compare harms from a legal activity with an illegal one.' This statement is something I am still trying to get my head around, as this is a significant part of what I am reviewing in this book. To me, a harm is a harm regardless of whether it's legal or illegal.

At the time of writing, I have no personal experience with this drug.

In the 1960s, it was proven highly beneficial for relationship therapy sessions. Psychologists discovered that MDMA provided a window of opportunity to get to the core of the problem quickly because it removed all conscious inhibitions. They said that a solution which would typically have taken six to nine months to achieve could be reached and managed with MDMA in just one sitting. If this drug weren't banned, imagine how many separated or unhappy couples could still be getting on well with each other and how much money they could have saved in ongoing therapy sessions. Oh, that would have meant the therapists would have lost their mass of mini-cash-cows.

Thankfully, in Switzerland, some therapists are now allowed to use MDMA within their sessions to help couples struggling in their relationships to find a quicker and more harmonious way forward, and more relationships have now been rescued.

At worst, couples seem to achieve a more harmonious separation and other potential benefits of reduced emotional and psychological stress on children and other family members. If this isn't an excellent side effect from the use of a psychedelic, then I don't know what is.

In Ayelet's book, *A Really Good Day*, she talks about how she and her husband privately use MDMA every couple of years to keep their relationship in full swing. What an excellent idea. In the reference section at the back of the book, I have included some extra fascinating info on how MDMA has been used for relationship therapy.

So, in summary, MDMA seems to be a very beneficial tool indeed for use in therapy, self-therapy, and to foster general feelings of well-being. Some risks should be considered, especially in conjunction with physical exertion. Here, it is vital to remain sensibly hydrated (UK: 0.6 (US: 0.4) litres or 1 pint per hour). MDMA can increase the heart rate slightly, so those with some heart issues may need to verify its suitability first.

Day 13: Almost 'The End'

Our parents were too big and powerful to blame, so we had to blame ourselves instead.

Complex PTSD: From Surviving to Thinking, *Pete Walker*

Dosage: Transition day
Physical Sensations: Over-sugared and jittery
Mood: Not so good
Conflict: None
Sleep: Disturbed
Work: Poor
Clarity of head: Needed my coffee today to function
Dark Thoughts: Dreamt of dying of a heart attack
Creativity: Not the best
Humour: Not a lot
Diet: Not brilliant
Daily Scale: 1

Last night's sleep isn't really what one calls good. The whole night, I dreamt that I was dying of different types of heart attacks. It's the first night in which I've had Dark Thoughts since I've started micro-dosing. I don't feel too motivated today; hence, I will write a short chapter.

Almost 'The End'

When I was having those near-nightly Dark Thoughts before I went through my NLP Breakthrough session several years ago, I had considered suicide due to several things not going quite to plan in my life. I knew it wasn't the right thing to do, but I didn't know how to escape my downward-spiralling situation. A good friend told me I would never know how my life story should end if I stepped out of the game too early.

I have always wanted to know how my life story will come to a close, so I pretended to myself that I had gone through with it and metaphorically died. It was a traumatic day for me, and I must have been quite messed up to simulate such a thing. I tried to use this as a new starting point in my life. I have two great friends who helped me through that difficult time, and I am still eternally grateful to them.

That is the past. Now, I need to focus on the future.

But not today. It's time to bring this to a close.

Day 14: No Contribution

The one who follows the crowd will get no further than the crowd... The one who walks alone will find himself in places no one has ever been.

Albert Einstein

Dosage: Normal day
Physical Sensations: Tired
Mood: Not good
Conflict: More with myself than anything else
Sleep: Slept through the night and woke up an hour later than normal
Work: Slow
Clarity of head: Muggy
Dark Thoughts: Dreamt of dying of a heart attack
Creativity: None
Humour: None
Diet: Poor
Daily Scale: 0

Due to disturbing Dark Thoughts concerning heart attacks, stroke and loss of movement I dreamt about through the night, my day today is in many respects not an illustrious one. Work is slow, and I am not motivated or inspired at all. My head isn't clear and free like it has been over the last couple of weeks.

I have now suffered from these Dark Thoughts two nights in a row, and I notice it is dragging me down again. Getting out of bed wasn't so easy this morning. Although I have made some progress with my work, it is weak and substandard, and I decided to delete it once I finished.

I isolate myself from all external contact today and withdraw into myself. As the evening approaches, lethargy dominates the scene. I even put off going to bed as I don't want to experience those nightmares again. It is nearly one in the morning before I finally go to bed with that same old dread of what's to come during the night, I had before I started micro-dosing.

Sorry, but that's all for today.

Day 15: NLP

Emotional flashbacks are sudden and often prolonged regressions to the overwhelming feeling-states of being an abused/abandoned child. These feeling states can include overwhelming fear, shame, alienation, rage, grief and depression. They also include unnecessary triggering of our fight/flight instincts.

Complex PTSD: From Surviving to Thinking, *Pete Walker*

Dosage: Micro-dose 100mg
Physical Sensations: Good
Mood: Okay
Conflict: None
Sleep: super. Woke up a little earlier than normal
Work: Productive
Clarity of head: Clear
Dark Thoughts: None
Creativity: Not really an opportunity to find out today
Humour: Good
Diet: I'm off the chocolate today
Daily Scale: 1++

Thankfully, no Dark Thoughts this last night.

A 0.1 gram (100mg) micro-dose seems perfect for me today. It kicks in within fifteen minutes of taking it without any dizzying rush to the head. My body is more alert today, and I have a more unobstructed view of what I must do for the rest of the day.

But today doesn't go as planned. I aim to start work on the third part of my trilogy. Instead, I will spring clean our apartment since my wife is away this week. Since there is a bit of furniture-lugging, I crack on with it and plan to have all the rooms clean before she comes home for the weekend.

My NLP Breakthrough Session

When I went through my traditional NLP (Neuro Linguistic Programming) Breakthrough session for a past issue a few years ago, it didn't settle my mental problems. Still, it did give me a tiny window to look through to realise there is a different world of reality out there.

This tiny peek into another reality kept niggling at me over the years until, after going into the hospital, almost dead, and coming out, fearing death, gave me something to hang on to until I started this experiment you are now reading.

If it hadn't been for that session, I wouldn't have started this experiment because I didn't think there was another version of reality as I was seeing it at the time.

On the one hand, it is a shame it took me a long time to get here; on the other, I wasn't ready. I don't think there is a time that is too late, even when we are old. I think it is worth living just one day free of that burden because we can say that what we went through helped us to get where we are.

I am still waiting for that day…

On that frustrating note, I think it's time to call it a day today.

Day 16: PTSD II, Traumatic Abuse and the Psychedelic Legal Movement

With psychedelics, if you're fortunate and breakthrough, you understand what is truly of value in life. Material, power, dominance, and territory have no value. People wouldn't fight wars, and the entire system would fall apart. People would become peaceful, loving citizens, not robots marching around in the dark with all their lights off.

Gary Fisher

Dosage: Micro-dose (100mg)
Physical Sensations: Good
Mood: Tired for the first couple of hours in the morning
Conflict: None
Sleep: Terrible – too much coffee yesterday
Work: Good.
Clarity of head: I know what I want to achieve today
Dark Thoughts: None, even though my heart was pounding through the night and kept me awake
Creativity: Good
Humour: Good
Diet: The start of a new day
Daily Scale: 2

…But the night didn't go well, and I accidentally made this a micro-dosing day instead of a transition day!

Yesterday, I drank coffee too late, which kept me awake until four in the morning. Today, I planned to experiment with a slightly higher dose to see the effect. Although I was up relatively early, I decided to wait until the next micro-dose day to be on the safe side. Three days isn't that long. But that doesn't stop me from achieving my goals today. My writing progressed, my research went well, and the day was productive.

PTSD II

Post Traumatic Stress Disorder (PTSD) is a relatively new name given to those who are suffering from personal traumatic events (as children and adults) and service personnel (military, police, emergency services, hospital staff, etc). PTSD affects nearly 8 million people in the EU alone. The saddest part of this is that around 18% of soldiers returning from Iraq and Afghanistan who have PTSD commit suicide.

That's more than those who die in combat! Talk about developing a war strategy...

The Difference Between PTSD and C-PTSD

PTSD is generally related to one-off events (accident, attack, surgery, etc). When PTSD refers to a series of two or more similar events happening over time (abuse, rape, war, etc), we generally speak about Complex-PTSD or C-PTSD for short. For ease of description throughout this book, I will use 'PTSD' to cover both.

PTSD categories cover and include various forms of physical/mental abuse experienced as a child/adult, an accident, surgery, war, natural events, a victim of an attack, verbal and psychological abuse, and anything that leaves the person permanently mentally affected in some way. PTSD is usually categorised in five levels (some institutions use four levels), depending on the severity of the disorder.

PTSD can affect people in different ways, ranging from not being able to socialise or communicate effectively and suffering anxiety when leaving home, having difficulties at work, experiencing extreme cases leading up to violent thoughts and outbursts.

Some sufferers tend to turn to prescription medication, alcohol, tobacco or other substances to help them through the day. Thus, in turn, can lead to lower self-esteem, a permanent sense of being in danger and being anxious when confronted with everyday events.

We know this is a complex, self-generating internal self-defence mechanism created by the brain shortly after the event. Over time, this defence process 'improves and grows' and becomes increasingly complex, to protect you.

We now know that the mind is a mighty machine that can create such defence mechanisms instantly. The quicker a traumatic event is treated after it happens, the higher the chances are of having a 'cleaner break' with minimal trace left behind.

In other words, the longer the destructive memory is left running, the more intense and complex it grows until it completely takes over a person's life, and the more prolonged and intense support is needed to be released.

For those who suffer in some way, it is essential to realise and accept that we have a lot of love, support and care from family and friends, although we may not be aware of it at the time. It can be a lonely world for a person living with PTSD. I know from my own experience.

There are different therapy and coaching techniques for dealing with PTSD, and the individual needs to find out what works best for them. Some effective treatment methods include trauma-focused therapy, eye movement desensitisation and reprocessing (EMDR), talk therapy and prolonged exposure. I've included several links at the back of the book on PTSD, which list more information on differing potential treatments.

This book is about using psychedelics in dealing with PTSD and how I dealt with my PTSD. However, if you think psychedelics aren't the right way forward for you, I would like to recommend two books to help you consider other options and to understand better what is happening in the brain. The first is related to childhood trauma and abuse, *Complex PTSD: From Surviving to Thriving* by Pete Walker.

I read this book after I had cracked my PTSD using psilocybin, and the book was helpful for me to understand what I had been going through. It also helped me to realise how messed up I had been in my thinking. I was then able to use this new knowledge to deal with specific 'gaps' in my life's experience, which left me unsure how to react in certain situations.

This book explained the nature of these gaps and helped me to gain a better understanding of life. If the book didn't show me what to do or how to be, it prompted me to search further to find out what is 'normal' and how to behave.

There have been several situations in which I have had to take a step back, assess, determine what to do, and then do it. Sometimes, I make the wrong decision, but I now know how to re-adjust to the situation appropriately. If a new problem is too much for me mentally, I can now calmly walk away without the old concerns constantly ticking in my mind instead of flipping out like I used to.

I think it is vital that we not sweep aside our traumatic past experiences and memories, as they shape who we are, give us unique qualities and resources, and provide a measure for future development.

The second book, *There Is No 'D' in PTSD* by Karl Smith. This book focuses primarily on PTSD within the services: military, police, emergency services, etc. and how to deal with traumatic situations experienced in the field. The book concentrates on the positive use of NLP tools in dealing with those past traumatic memories.

Suppose you are considering an NLP Breakthrough session or some other intense form of therapy. In that case, I recommend that you find a reputable Practitioner who knows how to deal with PTSD specifically and has worked with such clients before.

A good one is not so easy to find. If they promise you complete freedom, etc., after only one or two half-day sessions, you should consider whether this is for you. In reality, several intense sittings over a more extended period may be required, depending on the trauma and its effects.

However, judging from my experience and the feedback from other NLP experts, this support still needs to be forthcoming for a certain length of time following that first session, or at least until the client is sure how to respond and cope independently.

Before the use of psychedelics was banned, many countries, including the US, were finding great psychological benefits from psychedelic use for trauma sufferers. One shining example was the hugely beneficial work done by the British Dr Humphry Osmond while based in Canada.

Through his thorough research and astounding results with psychedelics on his most challenging patients, the government changed the status of LSD from 'experimental' to 'medicinal'.

LSD was used for treating alcoholics with a 50% first-time success rate, as well as for depression (the term PTSD was unknown then), with life-changing results. His widely recognised work included reworking children with autism with LSD so that these kids could integrate and lead a life.

Another doctor, Sidney Cohen, who carried out more LSD and mescaline experiments than anyone else, led him to define LSD as a very safe drug.

Many other scientists verified this clarification and successfully experimented with complex patients. He also understood that the client's setting needed to be a safe and stable environment in which they could understand what would happen to them during the therapy session. He also pointed out the importance of having a specialist nearby to provide guidance and support.

But it was the devastating work of Senator Thomas Dodd, who was responsible for the damaging propaganda that finally led to the ban on LSD. It's a great shame that so much progress over many years was disregarded. I suppose it was easier for Dodd to go down this more straightforward and unscientific path in getting it banned, rather than to work closely with leading scientists in finding the right and sensible way forward for the future health of humankind.

Unfortunately, the professional field had no choice but to go back to using some ancient technique similar to those first mental institutions by locking the patients away in decaying, depressing and damp cells. And let's not forget the autistic children who remain locked up within their inner world without having that chance of any mental freedom they once would have had.

Thankfully, however, we are now seeing an ever-increasing number of well-documented examples of personal experiences with psychedelics in which many have been able to overcome their mental and physical issues. Through such cases, we (the public) are starting to learn for ourselves where psychedelics can be truly helpful. It's these experiences that have helped me to take this massive step forward and to get results far beyond my wildest dreams.

Slowly, proper scientific research is being carried out once more, and in some countries, we are free to use psychedelics again. Once we have more conclusive results, we may be able to practically eliminate autism, addiction, alcoholism, depression, PTSD, etc, or at least give a fighting chance for those that need it instead of pumping them with Pharma drugs and their related side-effects. Let's hope so…

A Case in Point

At the time of going to print, the 'psychedelic legal movement' is gradually having success with cannabis, and fortunately, the laws are changing in the right direction. And if this can be achieved with cannabis, then surely it can be done with other psychedelics too. Canada, South America and Uruguay are leading the way with recreational and medical cannabis. Maybe Canada can lead the way again with the use of other psychedelics.

An excellent example of this problem is the English mother, Charlotte Caldwell, who recently had her son's cannabis oil confiscated by the Home Office due to its (unheated, thus non-psychedelic) THC content. Her son, Billy, suffers from around 100 epileptic fits per day, and THC is a natural substance available which can bring them under control (THC appears to be one of the most effective cannabinoids in fighting against epilepsy, cancer, as well as other illnesses too, as covered in another section).

Unfortunately, after the Home Office confiscated the poor boy's medication, Billy was rushed to the hospital after suffering a series of severe and life-threatening epileptic attacks. The government's problem was that traditional prescription medication was not helping him in any way, and he was reluctant to switch to alternative options, mainly when something contains THC.

Fortunately, a few days later, the Home Office relented after a public outcry, and now little Billy has his plant medication again. Thankfully, He is out of the hospital and back home with his family. THC saved his life and has stopped the epileptic fits. What is ironic about the Home Office's prohibitive stance is that the UK grows and exports about half of all medical cannabis used in the world today.

This family was lucky; there are still many children dying because international governments are still banning this powerful medication.

How politicians sleep at night knowing they have allowed so many children to die such a horrific death, I don't remember... I'd love to know that if it were their child suffering, would they allow it to die similarly, too, or would they be more proactive to change the law, so they could get something that works effectively?

This we may never know.

I hope that more such cases will bring our government to acknowledge the vast benefits that the cannabis plant has for our health. A British MP, William Hague, rightly said, 'The war on drugs has failed'. The government was never winning in the first place, but merely denying those patients who needed it for a chance of survival should surely be regarded as criminal behaviour and tantamount to torturing those who are suffering.

Day 17: Growing or Buying Mushrooms

Three hundred and fifty years ago, Shulgin notes, the Church proclaimed, 'The earth is the centre of the Universe, and anyone who says otherwise is a heretic.' Today, the government proclaims, 'All drugs that can expand consciousness are without medical or social justification, and anyone who uses them is a criminal.' In Galileo's time, the authorities said, 'We do not need to look through that mysterious contraption.' Now the government says, 'There is no need to taste those mysterious compounds.' In the past, the Church said, 'How dare you claim that the Earth is not the centre of the Universe?' Today, the government says, 'How dare you claim that an understanding of God is to be found in a white powder?'

Daniel Pinchbeck

Dosage: Transition Day
Physical Sensations: Good
Mood: Excellent
Conflict: None
Sleep: Good, and woke up earlier than normal
Work: Motivated and progressed with writing
Clarity of head: Clear
Dark Thoughts: None
Creativity: The Generation of material went well
Humour: Good
Diet: Nothing special to report
Daily Scale: 2+

I had quite a relaxed day today. I sorted out the apartment and rewrote some sections for this book. I also reflected a little more on what I want to learn from this experience and how I want to implement other changes in my life. Other than that, there is not a lot to report on today.

Growing Mushrooms

Growing the mushrooms with a pre-prepared substrate kit for this experiment was surprisingly easy. All I had to do was open the tub with the ready-grown substrate and drop it in the clear plastic bag provided. Next, I folded the opening and fixed it with the two large paper clips offered. Every couple of days, I needed to mist the sides of the bag to create enough moisture in the air for the mushrooms to grow.

The only other activity required was to air the bag for a few minutes each day and then close it up again. Then I patiently waited until they started growing. In less than a week, the first mushrooms were 'pinning'. The ideal time to harvest is just before the skirt rips open to release their spores. Several reports say they start to lose their potency once the spores drop. For me, this began to happen roughly seven days after the substrate had been pinned.

After one or two skirts had ripped, I harvested the more advanced ones and picked the following ripe mushrooms over the next couple of days until I had them all. The mushrooms were then dried in a dehydrator (max 40°C) to cracker-dry, ground to a fine and powdery consistency, and stored in an airtight jar in a cool, dark corner.

There are several ways to grow different types of psychedelic mushrooms from scratch, and I don't intend to cover them here. There are many good books on this topic. One I recommend for beginners is Virginia Haze and Dr K Mandrake; *The Psilocybin Mushroom Bible: The Definitive Guide to Growing and Using Magic Mushrooms*. This excellent book is a good starter guide and tells you all you need to know to grow your mushrooms, how to take care of them, how to prepare various drinks, and what to eat with them if you don't like the taste.

The Difference Between Mushroom Types

If you want to grow your mushrooms, I recommend the Psilocybe Cubensis family. Generally, it doesn't matter which one, although Penis Envy is the most potent in this family, which I wouldn't recommend for beginners. Mexican and Golden Teacher, for example, produce consistent results and are quick and easy to grow.

Where to Buy Kits

Maybe you don't have the chance to grow your mushrooms from scratch and would prefer to buy your pre-prepared substrate kit from a shop. However, this subject is not a topic I will cover in depth. If you want to investigate this, then check the options and legality for your country. There are a couple of good books on this subject on the market, and it might be a good idea to start with these and see if they help you.

Two of these are Joanne Hillyer's *Psilocybin – Magic Mushrooms for the Mind*, and Tom Williams' *A Quick Guide to Microdosing Psychedelics*. These show you how to work with the internet, make payments, etc. Otherwise, search the internet and find a legitimate supplier near you or check out some mushroom-related forums (I find *Shroomery* very helpful for all types of mushroom growing).

Buying a bag of grown and dried mushrooms from a drug dealer does have several drawbacks. Because they come from an underground market, there's no way of knowing their type, quality and purity. This inconsistency regarding purity is still a significant problem for all drugs sold on the black market. In the case of LSD, MDMA and other psychedelics, there are many documented cases of users suffering adverse reactions or even death, depending on the type of impurities used.

This inconsistency in quality is undoubtedly one argument in favour of legalising/decriminalising cannabis and other psychedelics. We will then know the product's quality, the supplier, the type, the strength, and how best to use it if we choose not to grow them ourselves. We can then relax and use them safely in our homes without risk of arrest. Precious health-service resources can subsequently be freed up without having to treat those victims who have procured contaminated drugs or have already turned to legal drugs with their associated issues.

Of course, as with everything, there is a small risk that one could have an adverse reaction to using psychedelics. People who experience a 'bad trip' could end up in the hospital, unsure of how to react. The total number of those who have difficulty with the trip's experience and end up in A&E is still significantly less than the numbers of those taken into hospital for alcohol poisoning or injuries suffered from drink-related accidents and violence. Paradoxically, one of the reasons given for the ban on psychedelics was that they were deemed to be a burden on our health system. Where is the logic here?

If we consider this scenario for a moment, that psychedelics were legal and bought in the open without fear of persecution, what effect could this have on society? From experience, we know that one of the immediate results is that it would drive down black-market demand, result in more affordable prices, give higher quality guarantees, improve availability and reduce the risk of impurities (other products added, artificial nutrients used, chemical crop sprays used, etc).

Not only that, but we would have the majority of the population who were suffering from some mental issue, free from problems and being a part of society again.

This law change, in turn, would free up already over-burdened police departments to focus on proper crime, reduce the burden on over-crowded prisons through unnecessary prosecutions and help reduce the number of family separations. At the same time, the government would earn a whopping regular tax payment from sales. Incidentally, the current worldwide black-market value of psychedelics was worth more than £67 billion per year in 2009, and it is growing each year. That's around £8 billion of potential tax governments worldwide are handing out to various drug barons instead of being ploughed back into society.

Then we, as taxpayers, need to add more money to this financial loss on the recurring costs of the failed war on drugs. This economic initiative alone in ending the war on drugs would save the UK taxpayer around £1.6 billion per year in extra payments.

If we consider that this failed war on drugs has gone on for the last 40 years, that represents a contribution by taxpayers in the UK alone of around £50 billion in total. And there is nothing to show for this immense amount of money the British people have been encouraged to hand over to the government without positive results. The only winners in this game are the drug barons, politicians and the banks.

In summary, by legalising psychedelics, we would pay less regular tax to our government, the streets would be safer and calmer, and the government and each respective town and city authority could receive additional finances from the psychedelic tax. This extra tax would have the knock-on effect of improving neighbourhoods, and the population's mental health would improve. Thus, it would be a win-win solution all around.

But that's not going to happen for a while.

Day 18: Addiction

We conclude that the present law on cannabis produces more harm than it prevents. It is costly in terms of time and resources of the criminal justice system, and especially of the police. It inevitably bears more heavily on young people in the streets of inner cities, who are also more likely to be from minority ethnic communities, and as such is inimical to police-community relations. It criminalises large numbers of otherwise law-abiding, mainly young, people to the detriment of their futures. It has become a proxy for the control of public order, and it inhibits accurate education about the relative risks of different drugs, including the risks of cannabis itself.

Police Foundation, UK (2000)

Dosage: Normal day
Physical Sensations: Relaxed
Mood: Good
Conflict: None
Sleep: Good
Work: Distributing marketing flyers in temperatures of -3°C
Clarity of head: Clear and positive
Dark Thoughts: None
Creativity: More of a practically motivated day
Humour: Except for the loss of feeling in my freezing fingers, otherwise good
Diet: slowly getting control of what I eat
Daily Scale: 2++

I feel good today and am in a practical frame of mind.

Spring is just around the corner (about six weeks away), and the sun is shining. So, I arrived home after distributing some flyers for my wife's business and continued cleaning the apartment. Thus, no real writing or anything creative is done today. The place looks so much better already. In the evening, I settled down with a couple of good films and ate a large packet of crisps and some butter biscuits with a couple of glasses of wine. Later, I went to bed with a bloated stomach and regretted eating that crap food.

LSD, Alcohol and Addiction Treatment

In a previous section, I mentioned that Canada had once changed the status of LSD from an experimental research drug to a therapeutic drug for use against autism in children, depression and alcoholism. This treatment was used successfully for many years until it was banned.

The use of LSD in treating alcohol addiction gained momentum following discussions between Dr Harvey Osmond and Dr Abram Hoffer. One commented that the LSD experience had a lot in common with the delirium tremens, agitations, delusions and hallucinations which are typical symptoms of severe alcohol withdrawal. Usually, such deliriums can be fatal, but they noted that those who survived them had the tendency to come out of the treatment with a transformed personality and remained sober.

This observation encouraged the two doctors to think along the lines that perhaps they could do the same by inducing such delirium tremens with LSD to invoke a similar transformational effect. Their first mini-experiment was with two heavy-duty alcoholics, and they stopped drinking immediately after their first and only LSD session.

Once the news of these significant results escaped, further success stories from other doctors started to crop up. It was noted that some patients needed a second session to free them from this addiction completely. Only a small percentage of subjects, however, remained alcoholics. Gradually, scientists started asking whether LSD could help against other psychological afflictions.

By the end of the 1950s, LSD was being used in the treatment of various illnesses, including neurosis, addiction, depression, psychosomatic illnesses, as well as for emotional and physical trauma. In England, LSD therapy was successfully used on ninety-four treatment-resistant patients, of whom sixty-one recovered fully or improved somewhat. Due to these impressive results, LSD gained kudos in the treatment of psychological ailments.

One of Osmond's alcoholic patients commented about his life-changing experience through the use of LSD; 'How can I explain the face, vile, repulsive and scaly, that I took by the hand into the depth of hell from whence it came and then gently removed that scaly thing from the face and took it by the hand up, up into the light and saw the face in all its God-given beauty?'

It's easy to forget that we all have some historical baggage we carry around with us from our childhood or an event in the past that causes us to react by trying to ease our conscience through judging those who have turned to alcohol or other drugs, or who have ended up homeless. In reality, I believe each of us is only one step away from being destitute, an addict of some kind or mentally troubled in some way and many cases, it's nearer than we like to think.

I think it is a crime that international governments have spread such disinformation regarding psychedelics to their nations, which has resulted in the banning of such beneficial programmes used in the past. The knock-on effect is that it has subsequently robbed sufferers of a chance to access proper life-changing treatments. I'm aware there are various recovery programmes available today that help many alcoholics and drug addicts. Still, they have never achieved the success rates achieved in the early international LSD treatment programmes.

The complicated and confusing reasons why the US banned psychedelic drugs are a long story and are beyond the scope of this book. However, I highly recommend Tom Schroder's book, *Acid Test*, which explains the battle scientists have had in working with and testing psychedelics. It also has some fascinating cases where psychedelics have helped people with life-restricting problems.

It's a well-written book that may help readers decide whether the US's propaganda was right. For an alternative perspective focusing on the demise of psychedelics through the behaviour of Leary and others towards psychedelics, I recommend reading Michael Pollan's interesting and well-researched book, *'How to Change Your Mind'*.

Historically, it could well be argued that international governments' decisions about what drugs should be banned seem to have been arbitrarily and inconsistently made, and they have been biased toward representing the interests of the larger pharmaceutical companies. The power of such industries appears to have led to extreme political lobbying, corruption, and a lack of governmental transparency. It is never openly revealed who receives what and from whom.

A good example is the political inconsistency of the case involving MP Victoria Atkins, the UK's drug minister. Her department, along with her approval, granted her husband, Paul Kenward, the right to grow a massive forty-five acres of cannabis under a government licence on UK land. And if that's not enough, her political stance, which she states in public and the House of Commons, is that cannabis should still be prohibited.

I suppose if this helps her husband earn a bit more for their future security from his international cannabis trade while the Joe public suffers, then I can understand her attitude by hindering further competition through her position within the British government. That doesn't mean I agree with her, though. Sadly, such double standards in political life today seem to be the norm rather than an exception.

An excellent historical example of the government's decision to ban certain drugs dates back to 1920, the year in which the prohibition of alcoholic consumption came into play in the United States. The official aim of this prohibition was to reduce crime and corruption, solve social problems, reduce the tax burden created by prisons and poorhouses, and improve health and hygiene in America. And yet this 'noble experiment' proved to be a miserable failure.

Although the consumption of alcohol fell at the beginning of prohibition, it subsequently increased later on. Alcohol became more dangerous to consume (impurities, government's poisoning of alcohol, etc.), and crime increased and became 'organised'. An adverse knock-on effect of banning alcohol was that the courts and prison systems were stretched to breaking point, and it unexpectedly removed a significant source of tax revenue, which led to significantly increased government spending.

And yet, those lessons learnt from this political disaster were not considered when it came to banning psychedelics. If only the government had researched the facts more thoroughly. And surely, we can rely on scientific reports supported by the government that psychedelics should be banned, can't we?

Ricaute's Report and the Banning of MDMA

A lot of controversy over the use of MDMA and its possible side-effects on humans was fuelled by the publication of the so-called 'Ricaute Report'. It was entitled *Severe Dopaminergic Neurotoxicity in Primates* and was based on a standard recreational dose regimen of MDMA. This report was featured in the leading journal 'Science' on 27th September 2002 by Dr George Ricaute and led to the banning of MDMA.

In Ricaute's report, it was stated that one of the five primates from each of two experimental groups had died, leading to the conclusion that MDMA can kill up to 20% of its users. Ricaute also claimed that even when not leading to death, taking MDMA could be linked to a severe risk of contracting Parkinson's disease and that severe or permanent brain damage could occur. Fortunately, many scientists were sceptical of these findings, which led to more independent investigations into the report. As questions about the results started, Ricaute responded with surprising answers.

Ricaute claimed that a bottle of Methamphetamine caused the deaths of both primates mislabelled as MDMA from the company producing the drug. Interestingly, the chemical company that labelled the bottles said they were never informed of the 'mistake' by Ricaute himself or by any member of his team. Finally, a whole collection of irregularities led Ricaute to formally retract his article in a new article published in 'Science' on September 12th, 2003.

Subsequently, it was also revealed that experiments in which MDMA had been administered to the primates were also deeply flawed. It turned out that these primates had received higher amounts of MDMA intravenously than a tablet would have contained. Not only is less MDMA absorbed into the body when taken as tablet form, but the amount that is injected would have been equivalent to taking a small handful of MDMA tablets in one go, which hardly any user in their right mind would ever do.

Another aspect was that the frequency at which MDMA was injected into the primates was significantly higher than a person would take in tablet form in an evening (usually once in an evening). Despite the shocking 'mistakes' made in these experiments that invalidated this paper, he continued to claim that there was a high risk of severe brain damage or death from taking MDMA.

Incidentally, typical deaths from MDMA have been consistently recorded as being less than 1% each year of total users. That's still less than taking aspirin and less than many other prescription medications on the market.

When properly used, many experts say this is a relatively safe and powerful drug that can give people their lives back, for example, people who are suffering from depression, PTSD, OCD, Tourette's and Asperger's syndromes and many more. At the back of the book, I have listed the potential benefits of the main psychedelics available.

I cannot find an answer to a question that comes to mind regarding the government's reports on safety. How many more government reports have been accepted and implemented, falsified, manipulated, or missing essential information? Are governments putting our lives at more risk than we realise?

I want to see more support and funding for research regarding the use of psychedelics. I also want to see the general public made more aware of the potential benefits and risks of all drugs, regardless of their legality, and the government should lead this. I also believe complete transparency is essential in all political debates when presenting official scientific reports.

Suppose a government representative or scientist stands behind a pharmaceutical company with finances paid into their pockets or through share ownership, etc., then this needs to be disclosed before discussions begin. That way, the right people can be brought together, and a balanced pro-and-con debate can take place with all the correct information on the table, which can then be investigated further. Once this information is verified, a non-biased person or board can make the right decisions for our future and that of our children.

I don't think these points above will ever happen in my time, if ever at all. Maybe I'm wrong, time will tell.

Day 19: Serotonin

The prestige of government has undoubtedly been lowered considerably by the Prohibition Law. For nothing is more destructive of respect for the government and the law of the land than passing laws which cannot be enforced. It is an open secret that the dangerous increase in crime in this country is closely connected with this.

Albert Einstein

Dosage: 1000mg (1g)
Physical Sensations: Good, light-headed
Mood: Good, relaxed
Conflict: None
Sleep: Good
Work: Spring cleaning!
Clarity of head: open and clear
Dark Thoughts: None
Creativity: Reflective
Humour: Good and relaxed
Diet: Dietary intake is under control
Daily Scale: 2++

In this experiment, I want to determine the effects of a light dose of 1 gram of psilocybin on me.

In preparing for my next five hours or so, I am wondering whether music would be good to hear, as I thoroughly enjoyed the 'Om' from my previous session. I have read about other experiences where some psychonauts have commented that it's better with music, although for others it is more of a distraction.

Ultimately, I decide I won't listen to anything and let my thoughts take me where they want to go. I also want to see if I have any good/bad experiences/sensations and how I will react to them now that I have upped my dose. I have also decided to focus on the points that bother me in the hope of helping me find out the root cause of these bad experiences, should they occur. So here goes.

I take 1g of dried mushrooms, make myself comfy and wait for the experience to begin. After about fifteen minutes, I start to notice its effects. First, there is some slight dizziness in my head. It's similar (but a little softer) to that room-spinning sensation I experienced when I reached my second cross-over threshold with alcohol. As this sensation increases, my coordination is becoming more erratic and unreliable. I decide to jump off the sofa and test my balance. Hmm, I need a bit more support than usual.

As I settle back down on the sofa, an array of colours and patterns dance around me, tuning their movement into my thoughts. As time passes, the patterns increase, slow down and then speed up, change colour, and swing in one direction and then in another. It is a beautiful show that I enjoy for about an hour.

In this session, I have no disturbing pictures, no 'bad' thoughts and notice no anxiety within me. I am relaxed and thoroughly enjoy it. Next, the sensory phase starts, and I feel every hair on my body, from head to toe, bristling away. For those who know me, it has been said that I could be the missing link between man and ape (I know, too much information), so the overall body sensation is pretty impressive. That tingling feeling washes over me in all directions and varying intensities. It is an incredible sensation. I notice my feet and body twitching as I lie on the sofa, like a dog does when you tickle a particular point on its belly.

After about three hours in, a spurt of energy comes from nowhere. I jump up thinking the ride is over and tootle off to the kitchen to make a pot of coffee. I bring it into the living room where I plan to enjoy it and reflect on what I have just gone through. Suddenly, I feel the urge to lie down again as another relaxing wave comes across me. Maybe five more minutes shut-eye and then I'll drink my coffee, or so I think.

Thirty minutes later, I sit up to pour my coffee, but the need to relax again is overpowering, so I leave my untouched steaming mug of coffee. By the time I do drink my lukewarm drink, my enthusiasm for it is no longer there, and I don't finish it.

Reflecting on this experience, I realise I need to improve my pre-trip preparation, and these are the goals I want from such a session. I'm now rather curious to know whether a higher dose than that which I have just taken would take me deeper than the superficial level I have just experienced, but I am not sure how much I would need to keep it safe.

A glass of water would have been good to have had nearby. I'm not the most stable on my feet at the best of times, and I was a bit shaky trying to get to the kitchen halfway through this experience to quench my thirst. And finally, I shall try to enjoy it more the next time. This time, I took it a little too seriously.

After attempting to drink some of my now tepid but strong coffee, I clean the apartment from top to bottom again (we now have an immaculate apartment). Then, I organised the food shopping for my wife's return home tomorrow after her week away. She now has a full fridge for her lunch when she comes back, as I'm not there when she arrives home.

I jump on the bike and head into the city eight hours after taking this dose. My pace and balance are good, and my reactions are quick. I would not have managed to get on the bike if I had tried to do this within the first few hours of taking psilocybin. It's as if an internal switch says, 'Ok, that's it. The trip is over. Now get on with your life.'

Would I do this again?

Yes. I love the feeling, the sensation, and the continual internal changing effects it has on me. I enjoy learning new things about myself. At the end of this session, I am relaxed and refreshed.

The drawback is that it takes quite a while to complete, and one needs plenty of time to make the most of a session. I had started at seven in the morning and finished at about one in the afternoon. I can't afford the luxury of doing this regularly.

Serotonin

Before any of us consider taking a psychedelic to get those neurons fired up, it may be helpful to understand what is happening in our brains when we do. The key neurotransmitter we discuss here is serotonin, which is linked to happiness. About 90% of our serotonin is produced in the gut, but this does not reach the brain. The key 10% is produced and used in the brain.

The effect serotonin has on the brain covers almost every area of our lives; sexual behaviour and appetite, aggression, cognitive functions, impulsiveness, pain, circadian rhythm, body temperature, sleep and memory. Serotonin is one of more than a hundred different types of neurotransmitters found in the brain.

Tryptophan is the primary building block of serotonin. The essential tryptophan sources are meat, cheese, dairy products and eggs. The problem is that eating more meat and dairy products doesn't mean that more converted serotonin will reach the brain because only tryptophan can cross the blood-brain barrier. Once tryptophan enters the brain, the enzymes convert it into serotonin 5-HT.

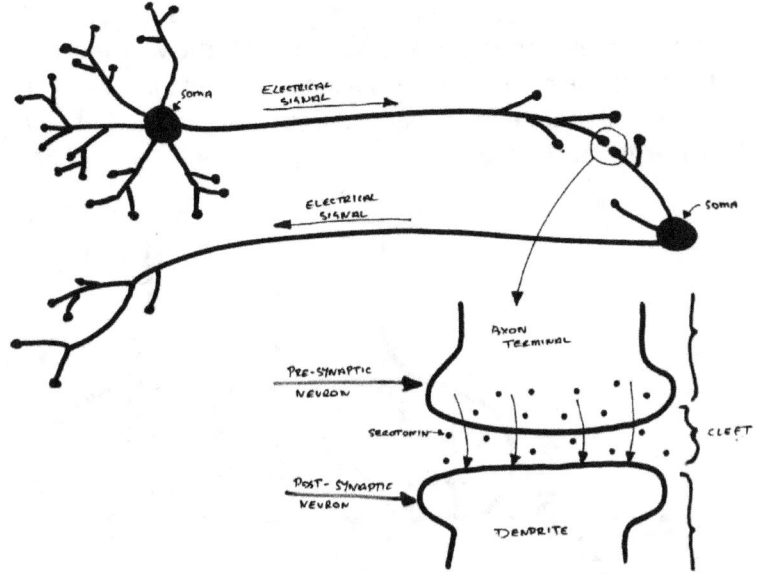

Figure 1: Serotonin travels from an Axon Terminal to the Dendrite through the Synaptic Cleft

When serotonin is created in the presynaptic neuron, it travels out by entering small sacs called vesicles. These then travel from the presynaptic membrane towards the synaptic cleft and wait there until the needed signal arrives. When a strong enough signal goes down the presynaptic nerve, the serotonin is released into the synaptic cleft (the gap between the presynaptic and the postsynaptic nerve).

Once free, the serotonin binds with receptors in the post-synaptic neuron, which then sends a signal down to the main body of the neuron. When enough signals are fired, they flow down the axon to its end terminal, thus causing a release of serotonin to stimulate the next neuron, and so on through its line of neurons until it reaches its endpoint.

Once a receptor has been activated, any spare serotonin that has not been used for neuron activation, it is either sent back into the presynaptic nerve to be re-used in the vesicle with other freshly made serotonin, or to a local glial cell that will absorb it, or it will be taken away from the synaptic cleft through extracellular fluid.

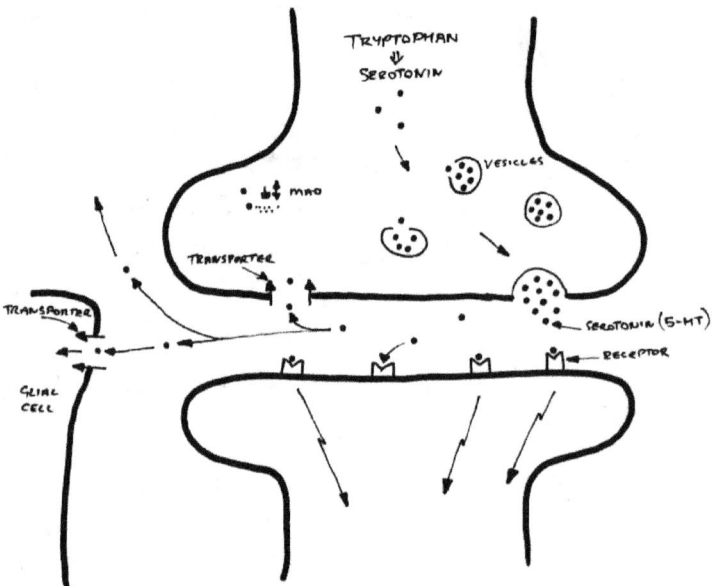

Figure 2: Serotonin leaves the vesicles and travels through the synaptic cleft to the receptor

Serotonin's Negative Feedback System

Because the brain can't produce large quantities of serotonin in one go, it can't release large amounts either. So, to ensure the right amount of serotonin is available, the serotonergic neurons need to regulate the amount released to protect themselves from overstimulation.

If there is too much serotonin in the synaptic cleft, then one problem that can occur is that the receptors become desensitised and don't allow serotonin to latch on. Another feedback control is with the auto-receptors outside the presynaptic neuron. These detect serotonin when enough receptors are around to latch onto them, thus regulating or 'throttling' new production if the serotonin count is too high.

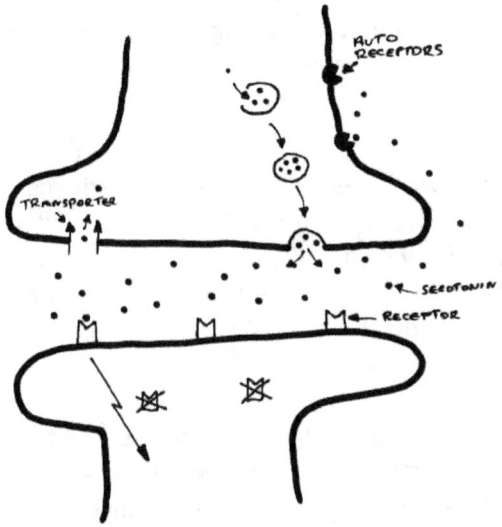

Figure 3: The negative-feedback system tracking the amount of available serotonin

Anti-Depressants and How They Work

Now that we have understood this, let's consider how antidepressants work. They come in two forms: SSRI and MAOI.

Several names, such as Zoloft, Prozac, and Lexapro, are SSRIs (Selective Serotonin Reuptake Inhibitors). They function by creating a blockage on the presynaptic membrane. Once this happens, serotonin cannot return to the presynaptic neuron and remains in the synaptic cleft, ready for latching onto available receptors. Remember, the more activity on the postsynaptic receptors, the greater the chance of a signal being sent to its presynaptic neuron, thus firing the next neuron and releasing more serotonin, etc.

MAOIs (Monoamine Oxidase Inhibitors) are an older form of antidepressant and are not used so often due to the high risk of debilitating side effects. MAOIs function by stopping the serotonin from being metabolised in the presynaptic neuron, thus effectively increasing the amount of serotonin available to latch onto the receptors.

How Psychedelics Affect the Brain

When we have a psychedelic experience with LSD, psilocybin, mescaline, etc, we can keep our executive functions working, meaning we can talk, think, go to the loo, etc. While some parts of our brain function normally, the activity in other areas of the brain comes to a virtual stop, making it an enjoyable experience for us.

Typically, signals travel from one point to another, but if this section of the neural highway is closed, the signals must take a different direction, like a road diversion. When these signals take new routes, we start to experience things differently.

The newly discovered Default Mode Network (DMN) is a key area that shuts down. The DMN functions similarly to a slideshow by showing us pictures at random from our past, of problems and arguments, of foodstuffs we have overeaten, etc. Once this switches off, our communication activity increases by around 1000x normal. DMN closure enables new networks to form, increasing communicative awareness and encouraging creativity, problem-solving and spiritual or therapeutic experiences.

MDMA

Ecstasy works differently from other psychedelics. It turns the whole process upside down. Not only that, it attracts a specific serotonin that is called $5\text{-}HT_{2A}$. This type of serotonin regulates our mood, anxieties, consciousness and schizophrenic behaviour. Instead of serotonin re-entering the presynaptic nerve, it remains in the synaptic cleft, and MDMA replicates serotonin using its molecules.

In the presynaptic neuron, the MDMA allows the serotonin to stay in the cytosol fluid instead of entering the vesicles. Due to the high serotonin available, the receptors are continuously being fired. Thus, we notice a fair amount of hyperactivity in our brain for 3 to 6 hours.

Fortunately, MDMA (as with other psychedelics) isn't physically addictive because serotonin levels need to rebalance themselves before MDMA can be effective again. In other words, several days of recovery are necessary before this experience can be successfully repeated.

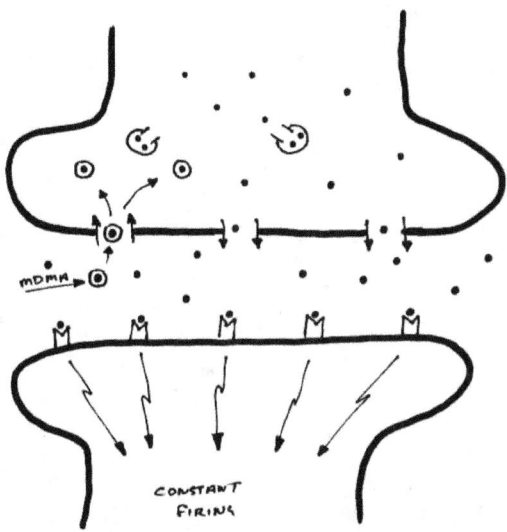

Figure 4: Effects of MDMA allow more serotonin to latch onto the receptors

For those who wish to read further about the effects of psychedelics on the brain, which helped me to understand this subject, I highly recommend a webpage called SapienSoup.com/serotonin. They have written further interesting articles related to psychedelics that are beyond the scope of this book.

Day 20: Psychedelic Access and the Water Pipe

It's not based on crime. The device that was used to recriminalise the black population was drugs. The drug wars are a fraud, a total fraud. They have nothing to do with drugs; the price of drugs doesn't change. What the drug war has succeeded in doing is to criminalise the poor. And the poor in the United States happen to be overwhelmingly black and Latino... Almost entirely, from the first moment, the orders given to the police as to how to deal with drugs were, 'You don't go into the suburbs and arrest the white stockbroker sniffing coke in the evening, but you do go into the ghettos, and if a kid has a joint in his pocket, you put him in jail.'

Noam Chomsky

Dosage: Transition Day
Physical Sensations: Relaxed
Mood: Good
Conflict: None
Sleep: Good
Work: More writing done today than in previous days
Clarity of head: Clear and focused
Dark Thoughts: None
Creativity: Better than first anticipated
Humour: Good, and probably a little cheeky with others today
Diet: I've avoided all the foods I want to avoid. Evening eating is a challenge, though
Daily Score: 2++

I slept well last night and am feeling refreshed after yesterday. My head is clear after my 1g light-dose experiment, and I look forward to the day. One of my original concerns was whether I would get addicted to psilocybin, but I feel I am in no rush to do this again. I still have much to process from yesterday, which will take me a while.

The day goes well. I write and research more than I had planned for this book today, and afterwards, I start to learn for a test for my German citizenship (a possible Brexit is looming over the Brits again as I write). Although I'm not a lover of revision, I have to say it went well today. I take a reasonable break and enjoy a good cup of coffee at a lovely place I enjoy visiting, just around the corner from where we live. I feel encouraged to leave the apartment for a while as the sun is shining and the birds are singing more actively today.

Besides that, there's not much to report except that I'm feeling relaxed and good. My head is clear, and I'm constructive in my thinking. My days are becoming increasingly productive. I'm lucky and grateful to have come across psychedelics. However, I wish I had discovered these benefits and started this experiment about 30 years earlier.

Access to Psychedelics

Which brings me to the question of who should have access to psychedelics. Should it belong to scientists (including therapists, etc.) or the general public? There seems to be an argument for both. Suppose there is a possibility of handling depression, PTSD, neurological illnesses, etc, with psychedelics so that we can live and have the inner strength we need without having to take long-term medication.

In that case, that surely is a good thing. I guess the Pharma companies will be screaming and jumping up and down that they would earn less money if psychedelics were used as replacements for many prescription drugs. But surely a person's health and quality of life is more important than the highest priority of selling prescription drugs with unsavoury side-effects to keep shareholders happy.

Death

Let's consider death. Most people fear dying, whether it's that last breath, the ultimate suffering from illness, life's regrets, unfulfilled wishes, dreams and aspirations lost on the wayside, etc, that plague us to the end. Not knowing how to come to terms with death can be a heavy burden for some of us to bear. Another option could be to take a therapeutic psychedelic dose, come to terms with where we are and what we've done (or haven't done) in our lives, help reassess some physical and mental pain and reflect on our past for what it was, so that we can leave this world with some tranquillity.

Many find it difficult to cope with the loss of someone close. Psychedelics can help to deal with that loss, to keep alive the great memories we have and to get on with life again. As you will read later, psychedelics helped me deal with the loss of my mother, who died a few years ago.

What about using psychedelics socially? Without repeating too much from what I have said before, one point I would like to reiterate is my belief that governments need to make sure that the proper information is made available to those who do decide to try psychedelics to avoid such tragic incidents as happened to the schoolgirl Leah Betts.

There is a lot of conflicting information out there (I know, I'm still fighting my way through it), which needs to be sorted out quickly. The public who want to use psychedelics will find a way of getting their hands on them regardless of what penalties are in place, either for social use or for private therapy, so isn't it better to get the correct information out there for the experimenters' health and safety as a first and foremost priority?

There's another aspect to consider, too. Our medical system is based on a cure rather than prevention. It means that the doctor is mainly there when you have a problem. Many of the 'cures' out there help to relieve or hide (mask) the problem, but as we have previously discussed, the conventional medical cures can also kill. We are now realising that cannabis is possibly fighting against cancer and many other illnesses without further damage to the body and mind, so why wait until we have cancer (or any other disease for that matter) before we fight back? Surely, it's better to hinder its chance of getting a foothold in the first place.

Before cannabis and hemp were banned, these plants were freely eaten as fodder by cattle (as well as other animals), which in turn flooded their milk with cannabinoids. The cows were milked, and the milk was drunk unpasteurised by us. The milk contained all the good and necessary bacteria in one complete product for our health.

What was terrific about this was that the good bacteria (ours and from the cow), along with the cannabinoids, were more than powerful enough to deal with many harmful bacteria in our gut. Pasteurisation, however, kills both good and bad bacteria, leaving milk toxic to us.

Oh, and cannabinoids are found in human milk from mothers breastfeeding their babies. This, incidentally, is missing in formula milk. It seems necessary for a child's health and a robust immune system.

Then we have many religions which are no longer allowed to use psychedelics openly, but which had previously played an influential role in ceremonies (Christianity, Judaism, various forms of Shamanism, etc). Couldn't the various religions reintroduce it into their proper roles again to allow the flocks (or, if it needs to be, just the ordained) to talk directly to their respective God again?

Wouldn't this be better than just talking about God like a permanently absent friend, like we currently do? Imagine going back to the days when psychedelics were used in defining religion by helping their followers to recognise their true spiritual potential and to meet their ultimate creator.

One point I haven't discussed is the resistance shown by the Pharma industry. If psychedelics were legally available on the market, the pharmaceutical industry would probably lose a significant amount of its profits, and several heavily financed medications that give massive profits for the shareholders might become virtually redundant.

Another potential knock-on effect would be that many doctors wouldn't get their bonus payments for the drugs they could have otherwise peddled, the customer (patient) queues in their practices would shrink, and they would probably have more time to assess their patients as real doctors should do by helping those who need it the most. Then there are the investors who could lose out, for example, the Mormon church has invested around $32 billion in the Pharma industry.

Again, I agree that we need an unbiased and official opinion on psychedelics, and more scientific testing needs to be carried out to verify all these new claims that are frequently popping up on the internet and in books, like this one. Up until the 1960s, before they were banned, medical and social research into the use of psychedelics was progressing in leaps and bounds.

Don't get me wrong, some modern medicines are essential. They saved my life, but in many everyday cases, I think it should be the last step for a doctor to consider when dealing with a customer's health issues and not the first. As with diet, so much misleading advice is being pushed around and marketed that people have become increasingly confused. This is where we should be able to rely on our doctor to provide clear and unbiased information.

I'm being utopic again, aren't I?

The Water-Pipe and Cigarettes

I had an experience that I had to fight against when I was at university. I don't smoke, but I don't have anything against it. As a non-smoker, I'm not a great fan of my clothes smelling of cigarettes after a night out, and I'm not too keen on smoky rooms either. However, I don't think I'm alone on that point. If someone wants to smoke, that's their life choice, not mine.

But first, the reason why I don't smoke.

When I was five years of age, my father was puffing away on a cigarette in the living room (this incident took place in 1972 when smoking was acceptable around kids), and he asked me if I wanted a go. Naturally, I agreed. He never showed me any love or trust, and I probably thought that agreeing to his suggestion might be a way of winning it. And, as a small child, I instinctively believed what he offered me would be good for me if it was good for him to do or use.

He held the cigarette to my lips, and I blew. Nothing happened. My father told me to suck on the light brown filter part. And I did with enthusiasm. I pulled the smoke to the very bottom of my little lungs. I coughed and spluttered and went through every colour of the rainbow. He supported me by laughing hard and loud as I struggled with my coughing fit.

Since then, I've never touched or wanted a cigarette again.

Fast-forward to university. One evening, after a fantastic meal a friend had cooked for a small group of us, he asked if we wanted to try his water pipe. After some consideration, I did. Other than that time as a child, the first thing I inhaled into my lungs wasn't government-approved air pollution.

I remember the cool vapour entering my lungs, which quickly gave me an internal euphoric dimension I had never experienced. Then I started laughing and laughing and laughing. We all did. It felt so good, and I felt so relaxed. It was something I desperately needed without realising it at the time.

Naturally, he said nothing about what we had 'smoked'. Instead, he just gave a wink and a wry smile. I would now hazard a guess that it was some cannabis Indica strain that was used. My problem began the next day as I wanted that sensation of escapism again. At the time, I knew nothing about water-pipes and even less about cannabis. But what I had to fight against every day for about a week was the urge to buy a packet of cigarettes.

A part of me thought I would get that much-needed relaxed sensation again, but another part of me knew otherwise; cigarettes don't give you that. Several times a day, I had walked into a newsagent, fought against the urge to buy a pack, turned around and left. After a week had passed, the yearning settled down, and I decided to keep away from all drugs. This decision included prescription drugs too, as it was also at the time when the government was pushing various anti-drug campaigns. Yeah, I was that gullible.

For me, those campaigns represented that if one type of drug is bad for you, then it must be the same for all drug types. I remember the TV programme *Grange Hill* and its 1980s 'say no!' campaign. I have vague recollections of the propaganda the government and the newspapers put out in the 1990s after the death of Leah Betts.

Day 21: Autism, Asperger's, Tourette's, Cancer and Chemotherapy

To the Daily Mail, stories about drugs not only sell papers, but ensure that policymakers will incur the wrath of nearly 2 million voters if they follow anything other than the newspaper's hard-line stance on illegal drugs. A former Mail journalist, who did not want to be named, said 'drugs are one of a hit-list of subjects given what she calls the 'Daily Mail treatment'. Stories are used to panic people.

Narcomania, *Max Daly and Steve Sampson*

Dosage: Normal Day
Physical Sensations: Good, relaxed
Mood: cheerful
Conflict: None
Sleep: Poor. Kept waking myself up with my snoring due to blocked sinuses
Work: Productive
Clarity of head: Clear, although I felt the start of a cold
Dark Thoughts: None
Creativity: Good and resourceful
Humour: Friendly and a little cheeky
Diet: Feel a little bloated, but no chocolate and bread today
Daily Scale: 2++

My energy levels are good today. Although I think I am starting to get a cold, I have planned most of my day before it has begun. The next challenge for me is to keep to it...

Writing and material research is very productive today, and I have found some answers to a couple of factual points that were niggling me and have updated this script accordingly. I have to say it has been an eye-opener for me as to what benefits these psychedelic substances can offer.

Here's a little of what I found out about Autism, Asperger's and Tourette's regarding the use of psychedelics. The benefits of psychedelics experienced for each syndrome are similar, and it appears psychedelics help significantly in all the cases in relieving them from some of their mental issues.

Further references and discussions are found at the back of this book. These are taken from open forums and reports, freely available to read on the internet and written by people who suffer from one of the three conditions.

Autism:
Using MDMA
'I guess it broke down barriers, is how I would describe it. Yeah, it felt like up until that point, I had always lived in a shell, like in a bubble. The way I isolated myself from people, and, yeah, I just tore that down, I said, 'There's no need for there to be a barrier.''

Using LSD
'Had symptoms, although more so hyper-empathy than no empathy, reclusiveness, compulsive/obsessive behaviour, social awkwardness, and language/speech issues. Psychedelics have helped me cure those almost entirely.'

Tourette's:
'I've got tourettes and that's one of the main reasons I started investigating psychedelics (the other being to banish the ghost of childhood night terrors). So far, from experience, I've learned:
- Weed helps the most. The only thing that keeps me sane daily.
- MDxx usually reduces tics unless a strong dose, then it has been known to trigger what appears to be a seizure.
- Acid seems to kill tics entirely during the trip and reduce them for up to a week after. Still, need to test the effects of a powerful dose.'

Asperger's:
'The pot is a huge win for me socially too, helped me chill the fuck out and start to realise what went on in conversation beyond just information.'

Here, I have selected a few comments, but there are many more, each telling similar stories. While the authenticity of all these descriptions cannot be guaranteed by reading them alone, these and other similar comments paint a consistently positive picture. As we see from the reviews above, each person has experimented with different doses and cycles to find which works best for them, and I'm pretty sure, based on my own experiences, that the first few attempts would have been a little hit-and-miss to begin with.

Some readers may see this as a risk, since the results may be unpredictable. However, no medicine gives 100% predictable results, which applies to all drugs, from aspirin to chemotherapy. If these drugs gave predictable results, cancer deaths would already be a thing of the past, and nobody would die from taking aspirin or other medicines.

Cancer and Chemotherapy
In the UK, based on NHS reports, the average survival rate covering 5 years of those treated for cancer using chemotherapy and other techniques is around 50% (2010), and this is significant progress considering the lower survival rates from cancer many years ago.

However, depending on the type of cancer, some of the survival rates over the same five-year period are nearly 97% for testicular cancer, 88.5% for thyroid cancer, 81% for Hodgkin's, 21% for stomach and almost 7% for pancreatic cancer, for example.

Unfortunately, one of the side effects of chemotherapy is that it can cause permanent damage to the body. It can kill the immune system and is known to be carcinogenic, meaning that secondary growth could occur. I appreciate that this conventional treatment has helped many people regain their feet, and I want to pay my respects to those who have endured such treatment. Yet, there may be an alternative without all the horrible side effects, and this is cannabis.

Survival rates from cancer using cannabis as medication are still officially unknown. However, more and more cases are becoming apparent from patients surviving cancer who were told by their doctor that there was nothing more that could be done for them using conventional therapies and that they should prepare for death in the forthcoming days or weeks.

Having to face such a horrific death sentence, several people living with cancer decided to take high doses of cannabis extract, such as Rick Simpson oil, also known as RSO, which is either self-made or bought on the internet.

Although this isn't FDA approved, more and more sufferers seem to be surviving and, in some cases, with all traces of cancer gone from the body. What is also remarkable is that there seem to be no side-effects; no killing of healthy cells, no permanent damage to the body, no extra suffering, no loss of hair, nails, etc, no organ damage and no risk of extra-cellular cancer growth.

Other potentially beneficial 'side-effects' seem to be a strengthened immune system, cleaner organs, a better outlook on life, no extra suffering, no sickness and no loss of appetite, etc. Incidentally, one of the key ingredients found in cannabis in fighting against cancer appears to be unheated (non-decarboxylated, thus non-trippy) and heated (therefore trippy) THC.

We may be wrong regarding the benefits of cannabis, but shouldn't we find out and carry out intensive and independent research on it to know for sure, rather than just relying on Big Pharma chemical concoctions?

I would also like to point out that an increasing number of people with cancer are now 'unofficially' combining cannabis therapy (smoking a joint about 15 minutes before treatment) with chemotherapy, and this appears to be helping sufferers to get through chemo sessions, overcoming sickness and getting their appetite back much quicker. I have included a range of links at the back of the book covering several of these aspects in more detail.

Many government scientists point to the fact that there is not enough known about specific drugs, or that the techniques used in the early days of science weren't thorough enough to allow cannabis to be used effectively. That may be true, but the same was true concerning the discovery of aspirin, pasteurisation and many other medical discoveries in their time, which have now been commercially accepted. Isn't there a bit of cherry-picking going on here?

We need only look at the amount of modern medication which has already been withdrawn from the market due to high death rates, serious side effects, etc. For me, it raises the question of whether modern medical research techniques are being carried out correctly if we are having so many drugs taken off the market. What is now being discovered in the field of psychedelic therapy appears to be a lot more convincing.

Simply put, if something works, shouldn't we research it further rather than have a blanket ban and force non-experts like me to carry out underground research?

The government says there's a high risk of death from taking psychedelics. Still, I would love to see the reports and figures that justify this statement, especially when various highly respected drug experts like David Nutt say the opposite. There are some deaths, but the numbers are so small, it should be embarrassing for politicians to even acknowledge them in comparison with the deaths from alcohol, tobacco and prescription medication. If the psychedelic substances are clean and not mixed with other (deadly) drugs or substances, as can be the case, then the risks would practically be eliminated.

As I have mentioned before, LSD was considered to be safe and was an approved therapy drug in Canada and other countries for many years. Can we assume that the political enforcers in banning psychedelics are trying to say that all these Canadians and other highly respected international scientists who have helped alcoholics, addicts and autistic kids recover and get their lives back, were wrong?

And then there are the supposed side effects of psychedelics, which, according to the government, cause permanent damage to a person's health. Well, the risk is also there with aspirin and many other Big Pharma prescription medications. So, what's the difference other than one being legal and the other not? Have you ever read what the risks are of what aspirin can do to us?

Here are a few of the side effects of Aspirin: coughing up brown blood, severe nausea, vomiting, fever, swelling, heartburn, headache, sleepiness, confusion, constipation, difficulties in breathing, fainting, changes in consciousness, anxiety, irregular heartbeat, panic, numbness, rapid breathing, restlessness, seizures, weight gain, and weakness in legs.

Oh, I almost forgot... and death. Consider, too, the risk the aspirin drug user is taking when using some machinery or driving. These side effects put not only themselves but others at risk as well.

This possible loss of life is treated as an acceptable risk by the general population since politicians have deemed these drugs legal. Am I standing out on a limb by saying that we should not consider this acceptable in how they are routinely dished out? Several thousand are going to die from Aspirin based on past statistics, and with this in mind, how do we know it's not going to be one of us? The problem is, we don't!

It was said that one of the early challenges with cannabis was measuring an exact dose of cannabinoids taken from the plant. Ripe cannabis plants vary in many aspects, giving slightly different concentrations of cannabinoids at harvest depending on how they are grown and what strain is used. But this is the same for all plants or animals grown, harvested or killed and mixed with other substances until the desired potency is achieved. Manufacturers do this daily with dairy milk, for example.

A bottle of milk is made up of white liquid derived from the milk of hundreds of cows, varying in nutrient levels from different farmers, and to achieve a consistent quality, water is added to balance it out. The downside is that if one cow has some illness or has taken antibiotics, etc., it enters the milk vat where it is mixed and contaminates the milk from healthy cows, which is then distributed to us without absolute protective mechanisms. Due to pasteurisation, most harmful and good bacteria are killed, and these dead bacterial bodies remain in the milk we drink, so we have to filter them out through our kidneys without any real health benefits. Eugh! I digress.

Nowadays, we know how to grow cannabis more effectively, consistently, and without the need for toxic chemicals. We can extract what is needed and measure it with greater accuracy.

We control this excellent substance more than other medications processed in factories worldwide. So, maybe there is a possibility of standardising cannabis extraction after all.

Phew, I think that's enough for today. Time for a break...

Day 22: Yoga and NLP Breakthrough

The paradox of the war on drugs is that the harder governments push the fight, the higher the drug prices become to compensate for the greater risks. That leads to larger profits for traffickers who avoid being punished.

Kevin Murphy

Dosage: Micro-dose 1mg
Physical Sensations: calm over my body
Mood: excellent
Conflict: none
Sleep: Super and slept through until the morning
Work: Very productive
Clarity of head: clear and focused
Dark Thoughts: None
Creativity: I am breaking new ground
Humour: Cheeky
Diet: No chocolate eaten today
Daily Scale: 2+++

After a two-month pause, I've just completed my Ashtanga yoga primary routine for the first time. I'm buzzing and have managed more work this morning than usual over a few days, and it's not even midday.

Around two months ago, I noticed a cold coming on and stopped doing yoga. It was a big mistake. After today's session, I now realise my body is weak and misaligned. If I do not do my yoga session for more than a few days, my stiff body aches when I resume. I have some physical challenges I've already mentioned, and yoga helps me a lot to keep me more aligned now that I've reached my fifties.

I work through the Primary Series except for the handstand linked with the Boat Posture (Navasana). I still can't manage Chakrasana (which I like to refer to as a backwards Vinyasa) without literally snapping my neck. I tend to complete the routine from memory or a 'Mysore' DVD.

NLP

A question comes to mind today. Through most of my adult life, I have suffered from depression and low self-esteem; in some rare moments, I have had occasional bouts of motivation, and I have had some great ideas. When I do, I usually start them with gusto, but rarely carry them through to the end.

And if I do, they always turn into a personal and mental battle, even if they do turn out well. When I look back on my life, I sometimes impress myself with what I have managed to achieve, yet I have terrible feelings about some super opportunities I have let slip through my fingers. In these last couple of days, I've had a remarkable experience, and I would like to continue this growth within me.

I **wish** I had had more of this mental balance and motivation I'm currently experiencing throughout my youth and early adult life. But I can't change the past and must find a way to accept it as part of my life's journey. But how?

Ah, back to the main question. Am I discovering a new me that will continue to develop into the future? Is the micro-dosing elevating this 'innate drive' in me, or am I merely reaching a level of natural maturity in my life, thus allowing me to mentally remove those doubts and insecurities that have hounded me all my life?

I think the micro-dosing is primarily responsible and not some sudden new bout of maturity. The changes are happening too quickly for it to be just a coincidence. But what about the effect NLP has had on me?

First, let's consider the situation where something has happened in our past, and the negative experience/trauma we suffered has significantly reshaped our lives. When this trauma occurs, it can instantly alter our thinking and life/reaction strategies by rewiring neurons in the brain. We can consider the key trauma when it first happened as the starting point, with a natural link to other lesser issues we have later in life.

Through NLP, we can remove some of these side issues by reworking the trauma and thus effectively rewiring the neurons in the brain. This process, however, does not work the other way around. If the problem worked on is not the key one but a related side issue, the situation tends to recur.

And that can only be good to know, can't it?

Day 23: Migraine, Ayahuasca and Religion I

If you get the message, hang up the phone. For psychedelic drugs are simply instruments, like microscopes, telescopes, and telephones. The biologist does not sit with his eye permanently glued to the microscope; he goes away and works on what he has seen.

Alan Watts

Dosage: Transition Day
Physical Sensations: Aching muscles from yoga – a great feeling!
Mood: Buoyant
Conflict: None
Sleep: Super
Work: Productive
Clarity of head: focused on writing and research
Dark Thoughts: None
Creativity:
Humour: Good
Diet: still no chocolate! Cool, eh!
Daily Scale: 2+++

Migraine and Headaches

While investigating what psychedelics could be used for, I notice today that people are using them against headaches and migraines.

Most of the feedback I have read about concerning the use of psilocybin as an antidote against migraines involved some sufferers taking an extra micro-dose as soon as they noticed the onset of one. Some sufferers found they needed to go just over the threshold for it to be effective, and that meant maybe a little lightness in the head without the real experience of an intense trip. They would rest for an hour or so, and then in many cases, the headache or migraine would disappear.

A young woman I read about needed to take a stronger, more potent dose of psilocybin to counteract the migraine once it had taken hold. I suppose the choice of either losing half her day due to the psychedelic effects and ridding herself of her migraine, or not being able to do anything for a day or two and having to suffer the side-effects of prescribed medication, was not a very difficult one for her to make.

There was one case I read about when a migraine sufferer took a significant over-the-threshold dose every four to five weeks regularly, and this helped to keep the once-recurring headaches at bay. That meant an intense psychedelic trip every month, but he found this a great way to relax and learn something about himself. His benefit was that he could then avoid prescription medicine and the associated side effects that he would have had to endure.

Although he had to sacrifice a good chunk of his day for this trip, he says he ended up with more free time due to the reduction in the frequency of those life-sapping migraines. I haven't mentioned any quantities here, because each person's needs are different, and it's essential to find out individually what best helps to achieve short, medium and longer-term goals.

One thing that seems clear and remains constant is that, of all the psychedelics available, psilocybin appears to be the best performer against most headaches and migraines.

Lucy, a friend of mine, regularly suffers from several migraines per week. However, she has been able to control them by carefully watching what she eats and drinks and being particularly careful while doing sport to ensure she doesn't jar her neck and shoulders from any awkward movements.

Lucy tells me her experience of a migraine attack she had yesterday. In the middle of the night, she woke up with a rapidly advancing migraine and considered taking one of her strong prescription migraine tablets. Those tablets tend to mess her up physically and mentally for a couple of days afterwards. She usually tries to wait as long as she can before taking one, hoping the migraine will disappear on its own, but it rarely does.

Then she remembered a discussion about the effects of psilocybin we had a few days earlier. She decided to take a slightly larger micro-dose (0.3g) than her normal micro-dose and settled down on the sofa at home. Within an hour, the migraine had eased up, and after another hour, it had disappeared completely, leaving her migraine-free for the rest of the day. She felt good and went back to her tasks like nothing had happened.

Is this just a one-off or a real solution for migraines? The simple answer is we will have to wait until her next migraine attack so that she can try this out again.

What Lucy loves about psilocybin is that she had none of the terrible side effects she usually has to fight against when she takes a migraine tablet for a couple of days afterwards. That means her liver, kidneys, lymph glands, etc, were not overworked or temporarily/ permanently damaged in any way.

Also, she didn't feel tired all day, which is another side effect she suffers from when taking medication. She could think clearly and progress with her day as usual. Her evening sleep was sound, and the worry of another migraine the next day was somewhat diminished.

There is one extra thing to add, I think, that is essential. On the internet, I found one guy who micro-doses with ayahuasca against his migraine, which gave similar results to psilocybin.

What Is Ayahuasca?

Ayahuasca is a brew made from Banisteriopsis Caapi – MAOI (MonoAmine Oxidase Inhibitors) and Psychotria Viridis (Chacruna) – DMT (N, N-Dimethyltryptamine). It's a traditional spiritual medicine used in ceremonies by the indigenous people of South America. The leaves contain DMT (a naturally produced neurotransmitter produced in the pineal gland), which is the psychedelic chemical. Although humans have a naturally occurring enzyme that neutralises its effect, MAOI counteracts this enzyme in turn, allowing the psychedelic to take effect on us.

Its medical benefits seem to be beneficial against depression, cancer, PTSD and other traumas. Another positive effect is that it helps to expand our consciousness by opening our minds and causing greater awareness.

From reading reports of those who have taken it, there seem to be no long-term side effects, except that the users are more relaxed afterwards, open to new ideas and live freer lives. However, the effects of Ayahuasca while in the system can be pretty intense, causing people to confront their greatest fears and to extract those personal demons that have hounded them for many years of their lives. One adverse side effect is that it can cause severe vomiting, although many participants say this is a necessary part of cleansing the body and mind.

For those interested in Ayahuasca, a fantastic book worth reading is about Mark Flaherty's inner battles and how he used Ayahuasca to get his life back on track, *Shedding the Layers – How Ayahuasca Saved More Than My Skin*. His struggle is inspirational, and his approach is helping me better understand what I want from psilocybin.

Religion I

Psychedelics have been actively used in religion for thousands of years and with significant influence until they were banned during the Medieval Inquisition onwards. It seems the main psychedelics used in various religions were psilocybin, ayahuasca, kava, cannabis, morning glory, peyote, wormwood and jimson weed. What I find interesting is that many Christians still condemn the use of psychedelics. However, when we review the texts of the Bible, for example, we find that psychedelics were often used to heal the sick, to 'get closer to God' and to anoint those into their sect to be in Oneness with God. According to the bible, it was classified as a potent medicine that had been used in antiquity, as well as in the lifetime of Jesus and others as an aid to performing 'miracle' work on the sick.

Many religions use and have used psychedelics for contacting their variously named God, Spirit, or Inner-Self for many years, and many individuals have reported having life-changing transcendental and mystical, religious or spiritual experiences through their use. Others have spoken about knowing their true self better, being able to make better decisions in life, dealing with a terminal illness, coming to terms with death, and finding out what God means to them.

For many, such experiences have been a revelation, a life-changing event that led to a closer relationship with their respective God. Who doesn't want to have taken that first necessary step in readiness for the next phase of their spiritual life journey?

Micro-dosing has undoubtedly helped me understand a little of my life journey, but it is not spiritual in any way. Previously, I would have said that my life journey had not been very interesting, and I hadn't progressed that far in life compared to others. However, that was until I discovered psychedelics. The one great lesson I have gained from taking a light psychedelic dose is that my life journey has actually been and is still amazing.

The thing is that I'm only just beginning to realise it. Firstly, I survived the first seven violent years of life in the brutal hands of my abusive and cowardly father and have, in some way, pushed on with my life through the support and guidance of my mother, which has helped me to fight against some of the demons my father gave me. And it's only now that I am beginning to realise who I am. It has been an arduous journey, yet the experiences I have accrued through my life have helped shape me, make me what I am, and start to appreciate that I am now at the beginning of a new phase in my life.

And on that positive note, I think it is time to come to a close.

Day 24: Who Should Micro-Dose and Why Ban Medical Testing?

Taking LSD was a profound experience, one of the most essential things in my life. LSD shows you that there's another side to the coin, and you can't remember it when it wears off, but you know it. It reinforced my sense of what was important—creating great things instead of making money, putting things back into the stream of history and of human consciousness as much as I could.

Steve Jobs

Dosage: Normal day
Physical Sensations: Good
Mood: good
Conflict: None
Sleep: Poor. I had a sugar rush around midnight due to an overdose on a home-made nut bar.
Work: productive and structured
Clarity of head: Clear and focused
Dark Thoughts: None
Creativity: Research on psychedelics pulls me further into this fascinating field
Humour: I'm feeling a little cheeky with others today
Diet: Not bad, except that I ate a lot yesterday. Still no chocolate
Daily Scale: 2+++

The sleepless night was due to a late sugar rush from overeating my homemade nut bar yesterday. I made these to replace the chocolate I'm addicted to, but I think that I need to stop this replacement, too, as they are addictive in their own right.

My research and writing are flowing this morning, with a wake-up to work start time of under 30 minutes. I love working early in the morning in preference to later in the day, so this suits me fine. Before I started this experiment, I would generally have needed at least an hour or two before I started working. Today, I am switched on quicker and feel more energised, which is putting me in the right mood for the rest of the day.

Today is a 'normal' day in my micro-dosing schedule, and I am just as charged up and energised as yesterday and the day before. My motivation has not been at this level for many years, and it's just wonderful.

Just one new negative thought that has crept in. I now have more summers behind me than in front of me. For the few months that have passed since my fiftieth birthday, I have been wrestling with the action-inhibiting thought that there's not much point in starting something new if I have the unwanted possibility of dying at some point soon.

The problem for all of us is that we don't know when we are going to die, and some never get the chance to reach the wonderfully ripe age of fifty. Maybe I should be grateful for that opportunity, but something within stops me from accepting it. I've still got many ideas about things I want to do and see, but the desire for real action is somewhat lacking. At some point, I hope I can get over this thing, whatever it holds me back.

In summary, over these last three weeks, I have felt more motivated, and carrying out this experiment has helped me find some direction in my life again. I still don't have the complete picture of myself, and maybe I never will, but I am beginning to like what I see and recognise. My desire to progress to the next level is slowly and steadily growing. I think micro-dosing is helping me with this, but I still have a long way to go before I reach my full motivational potential, if possible.

For Whom Could Micro-Dosing Be Suitable?

As I have realised from the positive information I've discovered in books and on the internet, pretty much everyone, the old, the young, the dying, the fit and the infirm could benefit from micro-dosing. However, there are some cautionary points to consider. For example, if you are on medication and/or suffer from schizophrenia, I would recommend checking first whether the medication you are on could react badly with psychedelics. I've written a more extensive section on this later in the book.

Generally, psychedelics are not physically addictive, although there are cases out there where people are mentally addicted to them. In many cases, it seems psychedelics can often prevent or alleviate addiction, for example, by weaning those off cocaine, heroin, alcohol and tobacco, if used properly. Some have managed to lose weight through micro-dosing, but this seems to be more of a positive side-effect than the main aim.

In some regions of Russia, mothers still make a child's dummy crafted from the abundance of wild cannabis leaves in the countryside for their babies to suckle on. The stuff grows like a weed over there, maybe that's because it is! Remember, if cannabis has not been heated up, then it has no psychedelic effects on humans, and the weed that grows in the wild has no real, definable THC-A content either. Interestingly, the chemicals in the Ruderalis plants seem to have nutritious and soothing effects on babies (and adults, too).

Psychedelics appear to be suitable for older people, too. Many people fear death (myself included), and micro-dosing (including light/regular/therapy dosing) can help to give us hope and inner strength to meet these fears. It has the potential to help people accept that their physical life will end, to experience being a part of God or whatever they believe in and to know this guide will welcome them on the other side with open arms when the time comes to leave this physical world. Surely, this alone is worth its weight in gold. Aldous Huxley did this with an injection of LSD on his deathbed and passed away peacefully. For Huxley, this seems equivalent to the Moksha of his utopian 'Island.' We may even suppose his desire was to experience his deathbed as the final enlightening and mystical state, an escape from the prison of individuality, a loss of self, a self-transcendental vision of the oneness and beauty of all this and a union with God/Spirit/Consciousness at that pivotal moment.

Additional problems many older people have include coping with restricted mobility and lower energy levels. What better way to enjoy one's final years than finding that little bit of extra pep to get back on one's feet again through micro-dosing? Even if one can't be as mobile as before, one could, at least, have a clearer mind and be more responsive to what is going on around them.

I have spoken briefly about depression on Day 14 and how psychedelics have helped to turn many lives around. For those who are suffering from a terminal illness with death rapidly approaching, it must be horrendous knowing that each moment could be the last, with unsolved issues remaining. Research carried out in the 1960s has shown that even taking a micro-dose just once a week started to have a positive effect on terminally ill patients after six months.

We have also seen that several people have successfully fought against depression through the use of psilocybin as a general pick-me-up using the three-day micro-dosing cycle I'm following here. Additional potential benefits for the depressed are taking a larger booster occasionally, followed by top-up micro-doses, which have led to significant quality improvements in their lives and with no adverse side-effects either.

Psychedelics have the potential to help the fit and healthy, too. It has been shown that cannabis (Sativa) improves physical performance. In WWII, soldiers were given cannabis and other psychedelics to provide them with extra endurance during their long marches. Soldiers have also used psychedelics before going into battle to reduce fear and increase confidence levels. If micro-dosing has such a powerful effect in war, imagine how it could help those involved in sport, endurance work and with arduous jobs. Micro-dosing is becoming increasingly prevalent within the business community and research establishments, and many modern-day pioneers have used it to achieve their current success: Steve Jobs being a notable example. More on this later.

Day 25: Religion II

And God said, 'Let the earth sprout vegetation, plants yielding seed, and fruit trees bearing fruit in which is their seed, each according to its kind, on the earth.' And it was so. The earth brought forth vegetation, plants yielding seed according to their kinds, and trees bearing fruit in which is their seed, each according to its kind. And God saw that it was good.

Genesis 1:11-12

Dosage: Micro-Dose 100mg
Physical Sensations: Calm and relaxed
Mood: Good
Conflict: None
Sleep: Wonderful
Work: Productive
Clarity of head: focused
Dark Thoughts: None
Creativity: Good
Humour: Good
Diet: stable
Daily Scale: 2+++

I had a brilliant night's sleep and woke up only once during the night. I haven't felt this refreshed in a long time, although I'm still not performing at my best. I know I still have a long way to go to realise my true potential, even at fifty. Nevertheless, it feels like an excellent and inspirational start to the day.

My morning begins well, and having been up for about twenty minutes, I am already working on my material. My writing is flowing, and the information I am finding concerning the potential benefits and uses of psychedelics is amazing.

Throughout the whole day, my mind is clear and focused. Knowing my thoughts aren't as scatty as usual is a lovely sensation. The one thing that goes wrong is that I eat a pack of Pringles and a packet of biscuits in the evening, and I (my stomach) feel terrible afterwards. Eurgh! Talk about an extreme and unenjoyable high from the sugar and processed chemicals rush.

I am irritable and tired in the evening, and I promptly go to bed. Now I expect those Dark Thoughts to come flooding back, showing me a multitude of ways of dying from a heart attack, and all those other horrible things that could physically debilitate my life, and deservedly so. I don't hold a lot of sympathy for myself this evening.

Religion II

In the Bible (Exodus 30:22-36), cannabis is called 'kaneh-bosem' (קְנֵה-בֹשֶׂם). It was mixed with oil to make an anointing agent (thus the expression of Jesus being the 'anointed one'). And if one looks carefully at religious art in books and on church walls, especially in Europe, it is possible to see the mushroom strongly linked to the early days of Christianity.

During the period after the medieval inquisition, those not involved with the church and caught using psychedelics were branded as witches or heathens, many of whom were then burned at the stake or drowned. From this time on, less and less is mentioned regarding the use of psychedelics within the Christian church or other main religions. Until recently, that is. Psychedelics are slowly making a comeback both in liberal Christian circles and in different religions internationally.

An experiment was conducted in the 1960s with twenty theology students in a church service. Ten of these students were given psilocybin, and the other ten a placebo. Of the ten students who took the psilocybin, they spoke about having experienced a magical, religious 'God revealing' experience in the service. Nine of the ten continued with their spiritual studies and were ordained. The second group of ten, who were given the placebo, didn't experience the same religious revelation, and none completed their religious studies. One of the nine ordained students who took psilocybin on that day is the respected religious scholar Huston Smith, who described the experience as 'God-revealing' and that it had been his first encounter with the other side.

Another study has been taking place with various religious leaders, including a Zen Buddhist, an Orthodox Jew, an Episcopal, a Presbyterian, and an Orthodox Christian. Their psychedelic feedback is helping scientists better understand the more profound philosophy of religion.

Although each individual's experience was unique, when their notes were compared, certain regular positive traits linked them together. Each of them, for example, noted a greater sense of self-worth, more love towards others, and a better understanding of cosmic love. This new understanding helped them to recalibrate their thoughts about life and the Universe.

Rather than putting this quote at the top of the page, I want to repeat the words here of Rabbi Zalman Schacter Shalomi concerning the achievement of deep religious understanding: 'It can be done with meditation. It can be done with sensory deprivation. It can be done in several ways. But I think the psychedelic path is sometimes the easiest way, and it doesn't require the long time that other approaches require.'

To summarise, one of the effects of psychedelics, which many people have, is an intense mystical and transcendental experience in which they appear to come face-to-face with God, receive a spiritual blessing and experience the revelations of a new spiritual inner-self. This effect has often led them to a greater self-conviction and strengthened their belief in their God and the afterlife. Another positive side-effect is that after such an experience, they tend to be less materialistic and egotistical.

We have seen that, whereas for many today there is a negative stigma surrounding the use of psychedelics, they have nevertheless been irrevocably bound to the development of many of the world's religions that we know today. Should we deny many believers the opportunities and chances of deepening their faith, inner growth and obtaining peace in the last days of their life with the help of psychedelics?

Or have I just gone beyond the religious pale?

Day 26: Caffeine and cannabis

My brain is only a receiver. In the Universe, there is a core from which we obtain knowledge, strength, and inspiration. I have not penetrated the secrets of this core, but I know that it exists.

Nikola Tesla

Dosage: Transition Day
Physical Sensations: Groggy
Mood: OK
Conflict: None
Sleep: Restless
Work: excellent
Clarity of head: a bit foggy
Dark Thoughts: None
Creativity: Good
Humour: OK
Diet: Bloated
Daily Scale: 2

I had to prise myself out of bed this morning, even though I was awake at my regular time. And here is something I haven't felt for a while: I am groggy, and I could readily lie down again to sleep.

Caffeine

Now, for the first sip of my desperately needed strong coffee, Ah, it slides down my throat and touches the soul, allowing me to start feeling human again. After searching through some material, I am reminded that Theresa May, the UK Prime Minister, signed a document in 2017 that banned all psychedelics except caffeine.

This is psychoactive, too, albeit a mild one. I'm curious about how she would explain her decision. Perhaps she is a psychedelic caffeine user too, so why ban something when one is into it oneself?

To find the official number of caffeine deaths wasn't easy, as many governments don't seem to record deaths by caffeine that clearly. After a bit of digging around, I found that around a thousand per year (US) and eighteen (UK) die yearly from this substance, which is in coffee, caffeinated soft and alcoholic drinks, caffeine tablets and caffeine powder. So, based on overdose death rates, we could say that legal caffeine is more lethal to us than illegal cannabis. I'm still not giving up my morning cuppa, though.

Cannabis

In previous chapters, I have mentioned that cannabis is a psychedelic and a relaxant and that most of us are already aware that it is widely smoked, eaten and drunk around the world, either for pleasure or for medicinal purposes. But there's a lot of unnecessary controversy about this durable plant. I've mentioned previously that the US managed to get this lovely herb internationally banned for practically the whole of the twentieth century, primarily due to the false propaganda stories created by Harry Anslinger.

Unfortunately, most other first-world countries were made to follow the US lead unquestioningly. For more information on Anslinger and how he almost single-handedly created a worldwide ban, I highly recommend reading Johann Hari's book, *Chasing the Scream*. What disgusted me is how Anslinger (also an active drug user and distributor of the very drugs he banned) created the basis for the illegal drug networks to become as powerful and as deadly as they are today.

However, before it was banned, cannabis was listed in the US Pharmacopoeia (a copy can be found on the internet) as an essential medicine treating over a hundred illnesses. It was, for example, the most used product against pain until aspirin was invented. And even today, cannabis is much safer and more effective than aspirin.

There are two parts to cannabis (not hemp) that should be considered: the trippy and the non-trippy bits. It is the THC content within cannabis that is categorised as the trippy part, but only once it is heated up (by decarboxylation). What happens in the heating process is that the acid molecule is burnt off (hence the popularity of smoking it), changing THC-A (non-trippy) to THC (trippy). Both THC and THC-A appear to have different but extensive ranges of medicinal properties.

Another beneficial extract from cannabis that can be legally bought in many countries is cannabidiol (CBD). This oil also changes from CBD-A to CBD when heated; when taken either way, it has zero trippy effect. Both forms of CBD have excellent medicinal properties, too. Currently, at the time of writing, governments are slowly realising it's possible to grow cannabis for its medicinal properties for the extraction of CBD without any traces of THC.

Medical cannabis, which contains THC, appears to have the most potential health properties and has been available legally in Canada for the last 20 years. In 2018, it was finally legalised for recreational use as well. It is also legal in South America. Other international governments, however, are proving slow to acknowledge the power of THC and CBD (amongst other cannabinoids) in the potential of fighting cancer and in treating different health issues.

The increasing pressure on these governments to legalise cannabis is continually growing from various pressure groups.

We live in an age of greater transparency, and it is becoming increasingly difficult for governments to hide behind the secret funding they are receiving and the misinformation politicians are disseminating to the public.

Cannabis Benefits

The list of potential benefits from cannabis seems to be plentiful. If you are considering using cannabis for illness, please check out on the internet which type of cannabis plant appears to be the most suitable for treating specific mental or physical health issues. Some of the significant benefits seem to be that it kills or slows down cancer cells, stops HIV from spreading further and in some cases eliminates it (as with raw coconut), helps against PTSD and mental health issues, fights against depression, relieves pain and helps with insomnia, treats nausea and vomiting. It also seems to help against epilepsy and Tourette's, Asperger's, concussion, preventing strokes, anxiety, stress, PMS, menopause, depression, glaucoma, arthritis, and much more.

The following is a summary list of some of the essential chemical agents found in cannabis and their potential therapeutic effects:

CBD: is anti-bacterial, inhibits cancer cell growth, is neuroprotective, promote bones growth, reduces seizures and convulsions, reduces blood sugar levels, reduces inflammation, reduces risk of artery blockage, reduces small intestine contractions, reduces vomiting and nausea, relieves pain, relieves anxiety, slows bacterial growth, tranquilises, treats psoriasis, is a vasorelaxant (reduces the tension in blood vessel walls).

CBD-A: reduces inflammation, inhibits cancer cells.

CBG: aids sleep, inhibits cancer cell growth, promotes bone growth, and slows bacterial growth.

CBG-A: reduces inflammation, relieves pain, and slows bacterial growth.

CBC: inhibits cancer cell growth, promotes bone growth, reduces inflammation, and relieves pain.

CBC-A: reduces inflammation and treats fungal infection.

Delta 9-THC-A: aids sleep, inhibits cancer cell growth, suppresses muscle spasms.

Delta 9-THC: reduces vomiting and nausea, relieves pain, stimulates appetite, suppresses muscle spasms.

Delta 8-THC: relieves pain.

THC-V: reduces convulsions and seizures, promotes bone growth.

The 'trippy' part of cannabis affects people in one of two ways - either making them sleepy or buzzing with energy. The Sativa strain is often used as an early-morning energiser, and it is the strain that soldiers took before marching into battle during various wars, or field workers took it at harvest time.

Conversely, the Indica strain is best taken in the evening to help you relax and to sleep well through the night. One point I found out, however, is that if Indica is taken for too long a period, it could make some of us lethargic, feel down and depressed.

Apart from being smoked, cannabis can be drunk and eaten too.

For those who can get a good collection of fresh buds and leaves to juice, this provides a great source of nutrients and the cannabinoids that are found in the plant. Also, because the plant isn't heated, there is no high; only healthy benefits. Before the ban, cannabis and hemp used to be found extensively in our food chain.

Various animals ate it using the cannabinoids for themselves and their offspring, and it was thus passed down to us through the food chain (milk and meat), providing humans with a safe and natural secondary source. Another option is to ferment it to make a Canna-bucha (based on Kombucha but made with cannabis), created and popularised by Colly Light.

A second option is to make cannabutter from the plant and use it for cooking or baking. Depending on the effect you want, the cannabis can either be heated (decarboxylated) or left unheated (or mixed).

A third option is to brew tea. A cup of Indica cannatea before going to bed or Sativa tea upon waking up is just what the doctor ordered. Or not, as the current case may be. In the evening, Indica relaxes the muscles, the heart rate slows down a little, and the blood pressure drops; racing thoughts in the mind slow down, and all this is followed by a night of deep and refreshing sleep.

Potential Risks

There seems to be a bit of conflict over what is safe and what is a risk regarding cannabis, and a lot of this stems from the propaganda pushed out by Anslinger. However, there seem to be a couple of health issues to be aware of.

Smoking: as with smoking tobacco, the NHS say there is a risk of lung disease and lung cancer if you mix it with tobacco. I assume that if tobacco isn't used, the risk isn't there. Another issue is that the NHS says it can cause cardiovascular disease and stroke. I know cannabis can increase the heart rate. So do sugar, bread and other carbs and apparently, they make the heart pump more aggressively and for longer due to thickening of the blood than with the effects of cannabis.

Driving: as with other drugs, the NHS say that driving under the influence of cannabis means you are more likely to be in an accident. I've come across a couple of conflicting reports regarding this, which say cannabis users tend to drive slower and, in certain circumstances, could be safer. We also need to consider that various prescription medication increases the risk of an accident. Still, no action seems to be ever taken against a medicated driver who has caused an accident. Is this just prosecuting those who break the law, rather than on the damage done to others, especially if we consider the amount of road rage, etc, occurring on our roads daily, for example?

Fertility and pregnancy: Again, the NHS says that this can interfere with sperm production and ovulation in males and females. Again, there seems to be conflicting information on this, too, which can help the unborn child. Maybe smoking cannabis isn't the best option when pregnant, especially with tobacco. Still, if there are health benefits with cannabis, as we've been discussing in this book. We know a mother's milk has cannabinoids in it; there are other ways to ingest cannabis that could be considered, if this is the case regarding health benefits.

Schizophrenia and Paranoia: These two are big subjects, and I have found them the most confusing. We know people can suffer paranoia from cannabis, especially if taken in massive amounts or for the first few times. For most people, this seems to disappear once we are used to assimilating the cannabinoids in our bodies again. The NHS says it can trigger schizophrenia in teens if used often, but again, there seems to be conflicting information out there that it helps to regulate schizophrenia.

Regarding schizophrenia, I have written a section on this subject near the end of the book on why this subject could be so confusing. Regarding those who suffer paranoia or other mental issues, there seems to be a couple of different reasons (I'm not eliminating this risk, but we still need a fuller understanding on this subject) and they could be diet related problems that are already causing brain imbalances and/or that they could have some mental issues that needs dealing with.

Another possibility is that we have some paranoia problems, which could be because we haven't taken cannabinoids since we were breast-fed. Maybe the brain is a little 'overwhelmed' with these beneficial chemicals. These possibilities and issues still need verification from further research.

Addiction: Getting addicted to cannabis (as is the case with many other legal and illegal substances, etc) is a risk. However, it seems to be more of a mental addiction rather than a physical addiction, as with heroin and cocaine, etc. One difference, thankfully, is that numbers appear to be very low in comparison to opiate addiction. I have addressed this a little deeper elsewhere in this book, that in many cases, an addiction to something is being used as an escapism from some issue or trauma in the past or present, or in escaping the anxiety of something that could happen in the future.

These people need some therapy to help them deal with those problems. Isn't this a fantastic marker (addiction) for our governments to say, 'one of our people has an issue, let's help and support them,' instead of pushing them to the fringes of society, to pump them with drugs and to leave them to suffer alone?

The NHS website lists a longer list of other potential issues. Still, these points above indicate one major problem I have highlighted several times: We don't know what all the effects of cannabis are, whether good or bad. This is an important indicator that we need to find out more about the truth through independent research.

Because our government doesn't support that research, the general public must find out based on 'hearsay' (just like I am doing here with psilocybin). The question arises with the NHS website at the time of writing: What have they based their information on? There are no references listed on their pages.

Is this because it is government-owned and they feel justified not to inform us of their references, or are they hiding behind non-informative political decisions? Don't get me wrong, I think the NHS does a cracking job with the political mess it has to deal with and the funding issues it suffers from, but we need to find a balance for our health and safety, and our governments are not doing that for us.

The Legalisation of cannabis

Let's consider the amount of money needed for the police to monitor and control the usage of this plant continually. We, as taxpayers, pay for this control in excessive taxes to the government to protect people against something many don't necessarily want to be protected from. Wouldn't it be better to legalise it, tax it, monitor its quality and content safety, know who the growers are and let us decide for ourselves if we want to try it? Governments can use this extra tax revenue for new projects, and the police will be freed to investigate proper crimes and put bobbies (police) back on the beat to make our streets safer again.

If we follow this (albeit simple) philosophy internationally, our world can only become calmer, happier and healthier. There would be less dependency on prescription drugs, alcohol and other addictive agents, which in turn, would significantly reduce unnecessary deaths, free up prisons, and so on.

This would have a substantial knock-on effect on the Big Pharma industry, hospitals, doctors' practices, and the sale of alcoholic beverages and prescription medicines. Because less alcohol is usually consumed when psychedelics are used, there will be less violence on the streets (alcohol related), fewer street/weapon attacks, fewer broken relationships, fewer hospital beds needed, etc. But if we consider our current government's attitude, this is a bad thing. It shouldn't be, it should be a good one.

Ah, and I almost forgot to mention, governments would have less opportunity to utilise their oft-used power-related weapon of fear on the general public to justify more taxes. Every government employs this human emotion to help explain its spending programmes and influence the masses to think in specific ways that benefit their policies.

Fear is sometimes used to hide other political agendas that are usually overlooked by the general public, and it shouldn't be. Fear funds wars, feeds terrorism and fosters distrust. Once psychedelics are legalised, maybe a lot of this fear becomes irrelevant, and future politicians need to think of different ways to manipulate the population to increase their popularity ratings. Or better still, they do their job representing the people. How do we know this?

When in the 1960s the US government needed to recruit soldiers for the Vietnam War, they were having problems with many civilians who had taken psychedelics and had gone through life-changing experiences. These psychedelic experiences led them to denounce the war, the military and its machinations. It's not difficult to imagine that if psychedelics had continued to be legal, the US would have become a more peace-loving country.

Day 27: Spirits and Their Physical Experiences

The potential of the psychedelic drugs to provide access to the interior Universe is, I believe, their most valuable property.

Alexander Shulgin

Dosage: Normal Day
Physical Sensations: light muscle ache
Mood: Good
Conflict: None
Sleep: Poor. Got to sleep around 2 am
Work: Good
Clarity of head: A little foggy first thing in the morning, but cleared up quickly.
Dark Thoughts: The first time in a while, and they gave me a restless sleep.
Creativity: Good
Humour: OK
Diet: I've put on weight
Daily Scale: 2++

Due to a late coffee yesterday, I had real trouble sleeping last night. I didn't need the late-afternoon coffee and made it without thinking. So, without further ado, it's time for my much-needed first morning coffee today.

In the middle of that restless night when I did finally fall asleep, I had dreamt of heart attacks, strokes, etc. I was relieved to be able to get out of bed and to start working as a distraction. Surprisingly, my start to the morning was pretty good, and I needed about half an hour to get my bearings before I could start working on this material.

It's slowly getting to the point where I'm nearing the end of this experiment, and I need to consider what happens next. Do I carry on micro-dosing with psilocybin? Is it worth it? And if I do, what do I track? The same things? And what would happen should I stop micro-dosing? Will I go back to my old self again? I hope not.

Lucy is micro-dosing too. She is, however, also paying close attention to the effect psilocybin is having on her migraines and her aching neck and shoulder muscles, which she has been suffering from for many years.

She said that she had taken a micro-dose that had taken her just over the threshold at around four in the morning. She settled in a comfy position on the sofa and waited to see what would happen. Lying on the couch in a particular position with lots of strategically placed cushions under her is a part of her routine, and it sometimes helps to prevent a migraine from progressing any further. And if she's lucky, she can avoid having to take a prescription anti-migraine tablet, but the threat remains throughout the day.

In this case, the pain reduced to an acceptable level within half an hour. Within two hours, she was back on her feet and pottering around with only a slight stiffness in her neck and shoulders. By the afternoon, her pain and migraine were gone, and she was absorbed in her work. Usually, with prescription anti-migraine tablets, some discomfort remains in her neck and shoulder after taking them, so this is a step in the right direction.

Due to the regularity of the migraines Lucy has had over her lifetime, she has often had to take prescription medication. She finds that they usually wear her down and make her feel miserable. However, over the last couple of weeks, she has noticed a big difference in her moods due to micro-dosing. She has discovered a new way of dealing with muscle pain and migraine without the unnecessary tiredness and uncomfortable side effects of prescription medication that remain with her for a couple of days. Will this prove to be a permanent solution for her? We hope so.

One small problem she has experienced a few times is very slight nausea from the psilocybin, which usually lasts for about half an hour. Thankfully, this doesn't bother her. Sometimes, before she started this experiment, she found that if a migraine was severe enough, the first anti-migraine prescription tablet didn't have any effect, so she would need to take another one a few hours later. The side effects of that double dose were not pleasant; they mentally knocked her out, and she usually had to take a day or two off from work to recover.

There are several side effects brought on by the anti-migraine medication she is usually prescribed. These include tingling of the skin, burning or prickly feeling or numbness, depression, bouts of dizziness, dry mouth, headaches(!), sickness and sleeplessness. The liver and kidneys must then work overtime to process those chemicals until the body has been cleared of toxic trace elements. As I understand, removing those elements from our system can take about three months.

Lucy intends to experiment further with psilocybin and monitor the results carefully to see the long-term effects. She is hopeful she will be able to avoid prescription medication entirely in the future.

The Spirit Having a Physical Experience

I find myself continually battling not just with my fear of dying, but also with the negative thoughts that arise within me when I reflect that at least the first half of my life has already passed me by. I have worked hard to overcome those debilitating thoughts that have plagued me most of my life with the help of various NLP techniques.

They have helped me, but it's still not enough. It seems psilocybin is taking this to the next level, helping me accept myself more for who I am, but it still isn't quite there.

When I die, I like to think that my subconscious will leave my body and later experience another experience as something else somewhere within this Universe. I want to believe that every living thing on this planet is special, that we fit together within a complete life-death cycle, and that we are somehow connected.

This developing belief leads me to ask: if I am a Spirit having a physical experience, how can I help my Spirit gain its best possible experience through me to face new challenges until my last living day? This way of thinking is helping to give me some perspective, thought and direction in my life. It gives me a focal point, and when I feel a lack of self-worth, I ask myself how I should channel my reactions and thoughts to gain more experience, which will support my Spirit for its next role in its forthcoming physical life.

And if I'm wrong. I will at least be able to say that I have lived my life the way I thought was right. Naturally, I have made mistakes and I will make more, but I aim to survive all my battle scars and their consequences until my life's natural end. I have to say, though, that I had had higher hopes that this psilocybin experiment would, by now, have confirmed my belief in the meaning of my life and that of my Spirit so that I could go forward with even more self-confidence in who and what I am.

Maybe there is only one current opinion regarding God, the Spirit, etc. in this world that is right, but which one? At worst, perhaps we have all completely misjudged it, and we are all wrong about what is waiting for us on the other side when we die. What then?

Day 28: LSD

LSD was an incredible experience. Not that I'm recommending it for anybody else, but for me, it hammered it home to me that reality was not a fixed thing. The reality we saw about us every day was one reality, and a valid one. However, there were others, different perspectives where different things had meaning, that were just as valid. That had a profound effect on me.

Alan Moore

Dosage: micro-dose: 110mg
Physical Sensations: Good
Mood: good
Conflict: None
Sleep: Good
Work: Productive
Clarity of head: clear
Dark Thoughts: None
Creativity: Not bad
Humour: Good
Diet: Still feeling a little bloated, but less so than yesterday
Daily Scale: 2++

My night's sleep was fantastic, and I slept right through. I woke up this morning feeling motivated for the day. I had no Dark Thoughts through the night, which makes a tremendous difference. I am amazed how quickly psilocybin has been able to change this, even after just a few days into the experiment. I am over the moon and don't have those Dark Thoughts as often as before.

Today is my last micro-dosing day in this 30-day experiment. Over time, I have increased the dosage in very gradual steps (from 100mg to 110mg), and I'm still okay. My only complaint is that I'm starting to dislike the taste of these dried mushrooms. There's a nasty bitterness to them that didn't bother me initially. It's only a minor complaint, and I can live with that.

With this slightly larger micro-dose, I still have my full coordination, although a very slight swimmy sensation in my head stays with me for about ten minutes. It's enough to notice, yet not enough to disrupt my thinking and coordination. I think I've found the optimal micro-dose for this batch of dried mushrooms.

LSD

I have said very little regarding LSD (LySergic acid Diethylamide) and its effects. So, let's get started on this fascinatingly powerful psychedelic.

It was Albert Hoffmann, a Swiss Chemist working in Basel, Switzerland, accidentally discovered LSD while searching for a blood stimulant (as a side note, it looks like the Greeks were using a type of LSD brew made from the same fungus in what was used in what we now call 'the Eleusinian mysteries' (15BCE to 4BCE).

This now-famous episode with the renowned scientist occurred on April 19, 1943, when Hoffmann revisited the product by taking what he thought was a threshold dose of 250μg (micrograms).

Yet, it was later discovered that the threshold dose is around 20μg. Within an hour, he experienced profound and sudden changes in perception. Feeling uncertain, Hoffmann asked his laboratory assistant to escort him as he cycled home, since driving motor vehicles in the evening during WWII was forbidden.

Hoffman described the sensation as '... affected by a remarkable restlessness, combined with a slight dizziness. At home, I lie down and sink into a not unpleasant, intoxicated-like condition, characterised by an extremely stimulated imagination. In a dreamlike state, with eyes closed (I found the daylight to be unpleasantly glaring), I perceived a continuous stream of fantastic pictures, extraordinary shapes with an intense, kaleidoscopic play of colours. After about two hours, this condition faded away.'

Later, its popularity grew due to the public's keen interest shown by psychologists using it in their therapy sessions for the life-changing results it seemed to have on many subjects. However, due to its growing reputation, LSD began to be used widely, yet unofficially distributed outside the scientific field and quickly became a common social drug.

One psychologist, Timothy Leary, encouraged US students to 'turn on, tune in and drop out'. This culture of LSD usage quickly grew internationally and, in the UK today, despite its ban, it is used more than in any other country in the world.

Although the US military tested its use as a tool of terror, it was quickly dropped from the programme. Apparently, all the subjects, after experiencing some anxiety and fear from not knowing what was happening to them, woke up the next day feeling a little shaken, but otherwise fine. Research also showed that US soldiers high on LSD became too unpredictable in warfare, and this put their men at a higher risk of being shot or killed by friendly fire.

LSD seems to be one of the most scientifically used, researched and documented of all psychedelics, and more is known about its effects than any other. In the mid-1960s, LSD was categorised as a Schedule I drug in the USA, meaning there was potential for its abuse and that it had no applications. Unfortunately, significant scientific medical progress was thereby halted in its tracks.

Micro-Dosing With LSD

Methods of micro-dosing using LSD are similar to those used with other psychedelics. Users are encouraged to stick to a 3-day cycle as follows until they understand its effects better. As with all psychedelics, the dosage needs to be kept under the threshold to enable one to remain physically and mentally active, alert, without any psychedelic effect. There are two ways to do this: either from a dropper bottle with LSD diluted in water or from tabs of blotting paper impregnated with LSD mixed in water.

A typical micro-dose for LSD is between 6 and 20 μg. LSD usually comes in 'tabs', which are little squares of blotting paper, aka 'blotters', which have been impregnated with the LSD. One 'tab' usually contains between 60μg and 120μg of LSD. Assuming 100μg to be a typical concentration value, then a micro-dose will be equivalent to about $1/16^{th}$ to $1/5^{th}$ of a tab.

This means that to micro-dose using tabs, these need to be cut into smaller squares, but it is pretty tricky to be exact with each piece. Another problem is that 1-tab should represent one drop of LSD, but as we have seen above, it is not always evenly distributed over the whole page.

The second option is to take LSD, which has been diluted in water from a dropper bottle. Because this is diluted in a specific amount of water, each drop equals around $1/10^{th}$ of a tab, which remains consistent with each drop. As with any psychedelic, if you feel unsure and still want to try it, it's always better to start with a smaller dose and then work your way up. This should help to determine whether you have any issues with it, as with any psychedelic or another type of drug, they may not be suitable for everyone.

Micro-dosing with LSD is hugely beneficial in the treatment of mental illnesses, including depression, PTSD, abuse, trauma, ADD/ADHD, mood disorders and addiction. Some benefits people gain from LSD micro-dosing are: creativity, more energy, better flow states, higher productivity, better focus, improved relationships, increased empathy, higher athletic coordination and stronger leadership development.

LSD (as with other psychedelics) encourages creativity, which is essential to many people in differing professions. Some prefer to remain below the threshold. However, most prefer to go above the threshold to achieve the best results. The effect stimulates the thought processes and improves problem-solving capabilities well beyond the norm.

Some famous people who have used LSD and other psychedelics with success include Steve Jobs, Aldous Huxley, Peter Matthiessen, Dr Andrew Weil, The Beatles, Ken Kesey, Jack Nicholson, Richard Feynman, Alejandro Jodorowsky, Francis Crick, Frances McDormand, Kary Mullis, Bill Gates, Doc Ellis, George Carlin, John Coltrane, Andre Previn, Carlos Santana, Alan Watts, Anthony Bourdain, Sam Harris, Susan Sarandon Phil Jackson, Cary Grant, Jim Morrison, Jean-Paul-Sartre, Jim Fadiman, to name a few.

Artists, musicians, authors, inventors, those working in high-stress environments, leaders, engineers, cooks, and many more are among those who lend themselves particularly well to LSD's creative benefits.

Micro-dosing with LSD and other psychedelics can also improve mental performance, concentration, studying, and sports performance by improving reaction times, finer muscle control, physical strength and better enhancement through physical training.

It is well-known that mental training is one of the most effective ways of quickly improving highly accurate physical performance. Yet, it seems that an even higher level of technical accuracy can be reached when mental training is combined with psychedelics. One such mental exercise might be, for example, learning to play a complicated piece of music and thereby improving one's finger technique on an instrument.

Also, when a piece of music is mentally rehearsed or practised with a psychedelic substance, the material can be absorbed much quicker, more specific nuances are noticed, and execution and performance significantly improve.

I was curious to find out how easy it would be to buy LSD on the internet within the EU. I quickly found 1P-LSD, but not LSD-25. Maybe it's one of those substances, like Ecstasy, that has to be bought from the local street dealer and needs to be tested for its purity before using it.

Several articles on the internet mention 1P-LSD as being the next best thing. This alternative option is legally available on the internet market pretty much internationally. Perhaps it is argued that 1P-LSD is not LSD until it is metabolised in the body, thus making it legal, and that it is a 'prodrug', meaning it is supposed to be used for research purposes only.

Hmm, maybe a project for the future.

Day 29: Lucy, Future Research and Illegality

Part of what psychedelics do is they decondition you from cultural values. This is what makes it such a political hot potato. Since all culture is a kind of con game, the most dangerous candy you can hand out is one which causes people to start questioning the rules of the game.

Terence McKenna

Dosage: Transition Day
Physical Sensations: OK
Mood: Good
Conflict: None
Sleep: Good
Work: Productive
Clarity of head: Clear
Dark Thoughts: Lots of death dreams through the night
Creativity: Good
Humour: Light
Diet: Stomach still feels bloated, but not so intensely
Daily Scale: 2+

Only today and tomorrow to go, and this experiment ends.

As of late, I have not had so many Dark Thoughts compared to the times before this experiment. Last night, though, I dreamt of several horrible deaths and re-lived my fears of not being alive for very much longer. Although I had a restless night and woke up early, I am nevertheless in a reasonably good mood, and my motivation is higher today compared to when I usually wake up after having those Dark Thoughts.

One reason could be that they occur less often. If, in the future, I can have them on average once or twice a week rather than the near-nightly event before I started this programme, then this is a significant step forward, and I can live with that.

Lucy

I spoke with Lucy later in the day. She tells me she took a light dose of 250mg earlier today, an amount that purposefully stepped over her threshold. Although Lucy doesn't have a migraine today, her stiff neck is bothering her. This muscle tension is usually linked to a specific point on her shoulder that can trigger a migraine later in the day. Within the hour, her neck muscles had relaxed enough, allowing the muscle pain to go away.

This result is something her anti-migraine medication never really managed. During her light trip, Lucy saw some colours and patterns when she closed her eyes and felt relaxed overall. She went through the philosophical (thinking/creative) phase and then experienced further relaxation. After five hours had passed, she went for a walk at a good pace and felt free and alive again.

After returning home, she found focusing on her projects much easier. She says the work she achieved that afternoon was outstanding, and she had accomplished more than usual in a shorter period. It's good to know I am not the only one.

Lucy experiences something else today. Despite the time of year and how warm it can be, she is like an ice cube. Lucy suffers from Raynaud's disease in her hands. Even in the summer, several fingers turn an off-yellow/white. She constantly freezes and must wear relatively warm clothes, even in summer. In winter, her hands are even colder than the Antarctic, and I guess her feet are too. I pity her partner when she needs them warming up at three in the morning.

Today, however, is different. After her dose, Lucy told me that the relaxation she experienced allowed the blood to flow to all her extremities so that she didn't need to put her gloves on for her walk. It is, incidentally, -7°C outside in Hamburg today. She's warm in winter! Is this coincidental, or is there a connection here with psilocybin?

After a bit of research, this is what I found out... Absolutely nothing. I've searched the internet and several medical and psychedelic books, and there is no experience documenting this reversal with the use of psychedelics. Or at least, I couldn't find anything. Is Lucy an exception, or is this the rule with psilocybin? She tells me that she still has warm hands and feet several hours later in the evening, and her muscles feel relaxed.

For the record, after about 10 months, Lucy says that her fingers have stopped turning white, they are much less sensitive to the cold, and she doesn't freeze as much as she did before. Is healing her Raynaud's disease all down to psilocybin or just a coincidence?

The Future

Psychedelic research is slowly progressing again, and new projects are beginning to take place internationally. I want to give a flavour of what is happening out there. Some institutions are looking for volunteers, and I've provided a link in the reference section at the back of the book should you wish for more information.

Let's start with MAPS (Multidisciplinary Association for Psychedelic Studies). This body is known for its research in psychedelics and is currently researching the use of psychedelics against cluster headaches. On their resource webpage for students, there is an extensive collection of information for those who want to either consider studying psychedelics or be a volunteer on a programme. This site has a wealth of information about psychedelics for those who wish to find out more.

The Heffter Research Institute is currently investigating the effects of psilocybin on cancer distress and addiction. This site has a wealth of information from leading medical and psychological experts.

The Beckley Foundation is conducting experiments to determine the effects on the brain. Their website contains a wealth of information, and you can get involved if you wish.

Several interesting articles published by Frontiers Media on their open-access scientific journals website, frontiersin.org, have dealt with issues involving, for example, the use of psychedelics and alcohol-dependent treatment.

The amount of available information is continuously growing and changing, and for those interested, these sites are truly worth investigating.

Day 30: Summary

Anger, depression, envy, sadness, fear, distrust, etc, are all, as usual, a part of life as bread and flowers and streets. Yet, they have become ubiquitously avoided and shameful human experiences.

Complex PTSD: From Surviving to Thinking, *Pete Walker*

Dosage: Normal Day
Physical Sensations: Relaxed
Mood: Good
Conflict: None
Sleep: Slept wonderfully through the night
Work: Productive
Clarity of head: Clear and focused
Dark Thoughts: None
Creativity: Good
Humour: Feeling cheeky
Diet: My weight has come down a little
Daily Scale: 2+++

Today is the last day of this 30-day experiment, and what an experience it has been for me. Last night, I slept undisturbed until the morning. I awoke as motivated and enthusiastic as on previous days and am eager to continue writing. This morning in Bremen, northern Germany, it is -7 °C, the sky is clear and blue, and everything is covered with a lovely layer of fresh white snow.

In fact, within twenty minutes of getting up, I am enjoying a cup of coffee, the stunning sun rising in the background, and I'm merrily typing away. There is something special about coming to the end of a project and reflecting on what has happened. I love what I have experienced and am eager to take this further, but I am still unsure how.

Summary

Now that I have completed this micro-dosing experiment, I would like to summarise the effects that the psilocybin has had on me over these 30 days, to determine how addicted I have become and how much it has messed up my life, according to government claims. Now I would like to run through each of these key markers and give you an idea of how they have changed me for the better, with no addiction and destruction of my life.

Physical Sensations: Before I started this experiment, I felt old and tired, despite being only fifty years old. However, micro-dosing shows that most of these aches and pains have eased up quickly. I have also mentioned before that I have a damaged leg and have problems walking barefoot on smooth, hard floors. When I don't take care of putting my foot down, it is as if I'm walking on drawing pins with each step.

My balance and agility suffer, and my heel often hurts. Trying to walk on 'dirty' floors with little bits of grit is next to impossible for me. Psilocybin has helped me slightly relieve the leg and foot pain, allowing me a bit of freedom barefoot, which is a great bonus.

Mood: There has been an improvement in my mood over these thirty days. My attitude has grown more consistent and balanced as the days have progressed, yet I know I still have a long way to go. I would say I am more cheerful within, and I am more relaxed with my wife and those around me. The positive knock-on effect is that we are both enjoying the new benefits. When meeting up with people, I am more at ease and can enjoy their company longer than before.

Conflict: The many conflicts I have had within myself from childhood to today have influenced me and made me who I am.

These include a lack of self-respect and self-belief, and a tendency to find issues with other things and other people's perceived problems that may not exist. Before I considered this project, my initial NLP Breakthrough session helped remove some destructive thoughts from within. However, I know that many of those issues still bother me and have remained untouched, and many inner conflicts remain.

I don't think about them so much now, and I think I can better control some of my emotions. This new focus is helping me to gain some self-respect. These small steps I've made are an incredible relief, yet there is still a long way to go.

Sleep: This is another unexpected gain. I sleep better and deeper than before, and have noticed the positive difference since I started micro-dosing. I occasionally wake up at night, but that's bladder-oriented chiefly and has, I think, more to do with advancing age than anything else. I like the often-optimistic feeling I have when waking up in the morning, getting up straight away and being more motivated for my day. This is not an everyday scenario, and the intensity is still inconsistent.

Work: I've struggled with my projects for a long while. I love writing, but more often than not, I have found it more of a battle than a pleasure. I ask myself how I've already released three (I now realise poorly written) fiction books onto the market. I know I'll never be a great fan of editing, but it has become a little easier this month. I also want to write, create something new, and achieve a higher standard.

And that's a great feeling I haven't had in a long time. I am now a little freer within myself, and that allows me to write with a more fluid style. Even around the house, I've been actively working through my To-Do List, which has remained stagnant for a long time. I'm even getting more organised in my office and work area. Again, this simple improvement is down to microdosing and is excellent progress for me.

Clarity of Head: One thing I have noticed from the first moment I took psilocybin is the calmness in my thoughts, and the stillness that comes over me is lovely. Even on transition and normal days, I experience some peace that has surprised me. It's not necessarily an all-day event, but I'm learning to enjoy it when possible. Even if I feel irritable somehow, it's not as extreme as before, if that makes sense. I love the ability to stop focusing on my inner battles and concentrate more on what's happening around me, even if it's only for a short time.

OK, I still have intense waves of fogginess and misdirection in my thoughts, and I can live with that much better. If you could have seen the pea-soup fog, thunderstorms and internal battles that were always raging within my head beforehand, you could say that I was in heaven before starting this 30-day experiment. Compared to what I am now going through, I'm in double-heaven. In reality, I still have a long journey to eradicate that fog.

Dark Thoughts: Before my NLP Breakthrough, my inner thoughts were a significant burden for me. If you were to ask me whether I was or am depressed, I don't know. I don't know how to assess and answer that. I've certainly experienced some real lows in my life (as most of us have at some point), and with the help of close friends and family, I have managed to claw my way out of some pretty deep and dark moments without the use of prescription drugs. Well, I think I have.. Maybe I have, and what feels like a fantastic release is still just scratching the surface of what is going on in my mind.

I have learned much from those dark moments, contributing to my inner growth. If I had been on medication, I think I would have had to live with the side effects that might have thrown me off-kilter into another spiralling dimension of misery. I would have never known if it were I or the side effects responsible for that new and possibly destructive direction in my life.

And if that had happened, then I might have gone from a partial to a total loss of control over my life. I believe I was right to reject medication for myself.

Although it took some time to get there, doing the NLP Breakthrough and understanding my PTSD for what it is was the best thing I could have done. That alone, in my opinion, has removed the need for medication. I opted for NLP on my initiative and was fortunate to have a skilled and highly respected practitioner to help me through it.

I now believe that an NLP Breakthrough can mark the start of a new life-changing experience, but it is not the complete solution. Psilocybin, so far, has enabled me to work through some other issues and understand them better than NLP could have given me.

Creativity: When I first started writing as a hobby, it was apparent that I still had much to learn about grammar, technique, and style, and I have since improved in these areas. Much of the material needed to be rewritten, gradually becoming less of a burden for me.

Now I can visualise scenes better, and my choice of words seems more powerful. It's not perfect, but it's better than before. I have been planning another book for a while now, but interestingly, I haven't known how to progress with the bulk of the story. That concept has been pretty much there for the last couple of days. Naturally, I still need to put in the details, but I enjoy doing this the most.

Humour: I have a dry sense of humour. Well, I am British. I liked to joke around and tease others when I was younger, but only with those I trusted. Then, my sense of humour started to desert me after a while as it went bitter and twisted. As I began to lose interest in things, I had less drive and dedication for those I participated in. Socially, it has always been that I need to leave once I have had enough of those people around me. It wasn't their fault, but mine. What I am trying to say here is that I am aware that my humour is a bit special, but I don't think I have noticed any improvement.

The one key person who I need around me is my wife. In this respect, we are both similar in that we don't need to constantly interact and rely on each other all day, allowing me to breathe freely within my private space. During these 30 days, because I have been able to approach things with more humour, it's also making my wife's time with me more enjoyable. And this is great for both of us.

Diet: Here's the interesting one. After the first 28 days of the 30-day experiment, I had put on weight. Over the last couple of days, however, I have lost that weight, and I am now back to my starting weight of thirty days ago. I want to think that is positive progress, but perhaps I'm a bit too optimistic here.

Was Micro-Dosing Right for Me?
Definitely!

Many areas of my life have changed over the past month due to micro-dosing. That change hasn't been drastic, but significant enough to take the edge off it and give me some of my old joie de vivre back. I now have some hope for the future. I intend to carry on micro-dosing at the same level as before. I plan to take the occasional higher dose for the wonderful experiences similar to those others have given me, and the positive mental and physical boost I receive from it.

Addiction: At the beginning of the book, I was curious to see whether I would get addicted to psilocybin. After 30 days, I still have no compulsion to take those higher doses regularly. I love the effect and benefits it has given me and the progress I have made in combating some of my inner demons by enabling me to continue my life's journey again. I have searched for examples of people getting physically addicted to psilocybin and can't find any, although some reports show that a few people may get mentally addicted to it.

It's these people who need help and to learn how to use psychedelics properly in dealing with their demons. I've searched for adverse health effects from psilocybin and can't find anything apart from a standard mushroom allergy. I can, however, find an abundance of those who have had significant and positive life-changing experiences from taking them.

Gateway to Harder Drugs and Other Issues: After carrying out a lot of searching on the internet, etc, I can't find anything to link psilocybin or other psychedelics to be a pathway to harder drugs, despite government claims (but I can't find their references either).

For those who have drifted to harder drugs, it appears that it is insignificant what they started with, whether it be coffee, cannabis, tobacco, alcohol, etc. As I have said above, it is these people who need the most help in dealing with those demons to help remove their addiction, as I hope this becomes a little clearer later in the book. I have found plenty of information stating that psychedelics ease dependence on drugs and alcohol, and in many cases lead to complete abstinence.

As the government says, I can't find anything to suggest that it can change or damage relationships. I have seen plenty of examples where couples have grown stronger and closer to each other with the use of psychedelics, however. Of course, as in any area of life, if two parties have strongly differing views on any subject, then it could drive them apart, but I can find no evidence that psychedelics lead to marital violence.

I have seen a lot of personal and some professional information about psychedelics helping those who had PTSD, trauma, Alzheimer's, Parkinson's multiple sclerosis, epilepsy, anxiety attacks, depression, ADHD, ADD, OCD, Autism, eating disorders, migraines, cluster headaches, rheumatism, arthritis, muscle diseases and muscle and joint pain, for example.

At this point in the experiment, I had intended to conclude the project and publish my findings. However, my research continued, and what I found unintentionally took me to the next stage in my life journey...

Sweet Spot No 1 – Guilt, Shame and Closure

We feel guilty for what we do. We feel shame for what we are.

Lewis B. Smedes

Since completing these last thirty days, I have read Tom Shroder's excellent book *Acid Test*, which has helped me consider new avenues of thinking and better understand the trials and tribulations psychedelics have endured since the 1960s. But it was his very last chapter that answered one question I hadn't been able to find an answer to.

That was the maximum amount of psilocybin required for the ultimate and safe trip to reach that Sweet Spot, or therapeutic, or spiritual experience, before stepping over that second threshold into the heroic dosing level. Incidentally, Tom Shroder states in his book that he learnt this from Roland Griffiths, the leading psilocybin researcher at Johns Hopkins.

My Sweet Spot

So, with some help from a calculator, I determined the ideal amount of my dried and ground psilocybe cubensis mushrooms. Roland and Tom say 20mg of psilocybin per 70kg bodyweight is required to reach the Sweet Spot. On average, we can say most dried psilocybin mushrooms contain about 6mg of psilocybin per gram, and the ones I have fit this perfectly.

This calculation gives a value of 3.6g of dried mushrooms with a content of nearly 23mg of psilocybin for my body weight. I weigh it out and add it to my scrambled eggs. This combination gives the eggs a slightly bitter, mushroomy flavour and is okay to eat. There's no way I could have eaten that amount of dried mushroom on its own, as I have grown to dislike the taste.

I decided to do this session alone without a sitter, drawing on my experience as an NLP coach. I should be able to stay grounded throughout. I have my mobile next to me, in case I lose the plot at any time. Being alone guarantees no disturbances, no external questions or comments coming at me, etc., and I can let my subconscious drive me the way it needs to so it can give me the answers I need to my problem.

I have some pre-prepared questions that I hope to find a solution to during this session. The one person I still miss the most in my life is my Mum, who died several years ago. Mum had to endure the crippling effects of MS (multiple sclerosis) in the last years of her life. Her battle against that disease over the fourteen years was immense. Her suffering tore me apart, and I still have a lot of problems dealing with it.

I have always felt I had never supported her the way I should or could have, especially when I consider the turmoil she went through in her early years from the abuse she suffered at the hands of her violent husband, in trying to protect me when I was a baby and small child. If it wasn't for my sister, other family members and friends, I don't even want to think about how I would not have dealt with Mum's illness.

So, from this session, I don't need forgiveness or pity. I need closure, though, and I am willing to take all the burdens on my shoulders to get it.

About fifteen minutes after eating the mushrooms with the eggs, I began to feel the effects of the mushrooms. I quickly realised that those just 'over-the-threshold' experiences I had during the 30-day experiment were light, gentle, playful, and nothing more than a bit of escapism from the real world.

The sensation I now have is a whole body and mind experience, and I am already in awe of its first effects on me. To begin with,

I am on a smooth and enjoyable kaleidoscopic journey as I notice my muscles and mind begin to relax. I decide to go to the safety of my bed and experience whatever is to happen to me from there.

Now, in my psychedelic state, I find myself slowly and gradually 'linking up' to this cancer I have felt for many years within my stomach. I am witnessing scenes inside my belly as I visit various places one after another, where I had endured horrible things as a child. There is a snippet of the living room, my bedroom, my parents' bedroom, the bathroom, the kitchen, the back and front garden.

I hear the fights, slaps, punches, shouting, breaking of bones, pleading and crying in these scenes as if they were happening. Strong feelings of guilt and shame engulf me, destroying any remaining hope of closure I have left within me.

I revisit these scenes, such that each of those painful experiences is reworked and processed and twisted and pulled apart one after another. Then I try to put them back together differently, but it makes no difference. My guilt and shame remain as they were before.

The next stage is where the scenery changes entirely in an instant. I meet someone I know and highly respect personally in the real world, and I bond spiritually with them for several minutes. We are linking up with each other, a bit like two parts of a lock fitting together and becoming one. And suddenly, I realise that this person's role is that of the gatekeeper on the other side. I hear and feel a 'click' and another world opens.

I enter the Universe.

And as I am floating in the Universe, those past problems, the abuse, the torment, the guilt, and the shame dissolve within an instant. Parts of my life suddenly start to make sense to me. Here, I realise how inadequate our language can be to describe such experiences as this.

Some of my life's problems float around me, and I see (not feel) the emotions because they are disconnected from me. I know it doesn't make sense, but that's the best way I can describe it. In an instant, all those negative sensations around me disappear, leaving me with a sense of tranquillity.

The next sensation I experience is that I am becoming a part of the Universe. When I look around at this vastness, I see the roots of the souls of all the living beings in the real world, but many of these roots barely touch the Universe's vast potential.

Occasionally, I see a person's root that has deeply bonded with the Universe, yet I don't know who it is, and I can't determine how they are affected by it. Interestingly, I can see the roots of plants, birds and animals, and most of these are connected to the Universe. Then I realise that my roots are finally planted into the Universe and begin to grow and penetrate deeper into the welcoming Universe.

I also feel my mum around me. I wanted to see her and communicate with her in some way to apologise for letting her down and not being there for her, but this experience is far different and more meaningful than I imagined it could be. Her spirit is all around me, supporting me in absolute love and understanding.

I notice other spirits flying around me, the people I now realise were once important to me before they died. Suddenly, those related past traumas and problems are gone. In my mind, I am far more relaxed and more confident.

I've led a lonely life in many respects and tried to solve most of my problems alone. After fifty years of trying, it has finally become clear that this old way is not working. Yet, here I am in the Universe! Suddenly, I can breathe without restriction and discard some of my limiting and confusing perceptions of my self-identity.

My loneliness has given way to feelings of great contentment. A unity now holds me together with others a little more. This bonding with others is something my sister could always do, which I have always struggled with. I am so grateful that she was able to give Mum the love and support in her most difficult moments that I couldn't provide.

At this moment, I understand them both much better, and they're not judging me. Nobody is, and they never have. I only realised it at this moment. Their family love has always been unconditional. It's now clear they've understood me better than I have ever understood myself over all these years.

This last part of the process has taken about an hour, and I am urged to shower. So far, I have completed around four hours of this Sweet Spot journey. Over the last few days, I have read about Wim Hof and his breathing techniques.

Wim says that we all have a relationship with the cold and that it can help heal us from the inside. I take a shower and enjoy the feeling of the hot water pouring over me. I swing the shower temperature lever to cold, manage about an uncontrolled second, scream in shock and yank the lever back to hot. Wim talks about steady breathing, like Bastrika in Pranayama; the lungs are filled up and quickly collapse to force the stale air out.

So, I breathe deeply into my lungs through my nose and allow the stale air to flow out of my mouth, nice and steady. It is an incredible sensation, and with the sound of water cascading over my head, it becomes suddenly amazing. After about thirty breaths, I swing the lever to cold and that icy water hits me from top to bottom.

I breathe steadily and slowly, so I recognise myself opening up from the inside. Then suddenly, I experience a massive emotional release, which is exhilarating. I do this for about five minutes, under the freezing water, which is invigorating. I now understand why this is so important to our health and well-being. I switch off the ice-cold water and am feeling alive and free, truly free from those shackles I have carried for most of my life (I would like to add that I have tried that same cold shower several times since and to date, I have managed no more than fifteen seconds).

It's now six hours since I took the psilocybin. I settle down and drink a cup of tea, reflecting on what I have just gone through. I will contemplate this experience for the next few days, if not in the coming weeks. And I still sense this personal connection with the Universe.

Maybe I still have some psilocybin flowing through my system. I don't know. I reflect upon the difference I have experienced mentally between my NLP Breakthrough and this new experience with psilocybin. Both are fantastic and beneficial experiences. At this point, a question comes to mind: was what I have just experienced real or merely a collage of images and memories from my past?

The journey I described above is similar to having many dreams packed together. I'm not quite sure of the exact sequence of events anymore, nor how those lifelong issues came to a closure; they just did. Many things were happening in my mind at lightning speed, so much happened so quickly that I could not remember any of the details. My challenge here is trying to put this experience into words.

I have reached a closure regarding my Mum, and I now notice her presence in a way I could never have anticipated. Her birthday is in a couple of weeks, which is always a hard time for me, and I'll know better when it has passed...

Note: Mum's birthday has since come and gone, and I felt fine and had tremendous love for her, reflecting on my memories of her. I am still sad she is no longer here, but for the first time, I am now free from that ever-growing feeling of guilt and shame which had burdened me.

In his interesting book *The Psychedelic Future of the Mind*, Thomas B. Roberts proposes various theories about what could be happening in these sessions. One of these is that we create our world in our minds, enabling us to encounter the Universe. When we do this, we use a personal gateway to access the universe, which is made possible by using specific plants we naturally find on our planet.

Another point is that all those experiences from our forefathers we have gathered over time are stored within our memory banks and in our genes, thus giving us a sizeable and generational history to reflect upon. But what about my experience of the Universe? Did I (and some of my forefathers) witness that? Does it really exist? And who does that make crazy, those who deny and disbelieve it or have experienced it? Real or not, it has profoundly affected me and, judging by how I feel, probably a lasting one too.

The Next Day

By the evening of the same day I carried out the Sweet Spot experiment, I was tired and was more than happy to go to bed early. This tiredness is more than I imagined, and I would not be ready for sleep until late or early the next morning. When I did go to bed, I slept like a contented baby through the night. I remember dreaming, yet the dreams were so light and free that I couldn't remember their details. I had no Dark Thoughts through the night whatsoever. When I woke up this morning, I felt light and refreshed, and I just wanted to get up and get on with the day.

As I sit here typing this, I notice that the tension in my chest for several years has gone away. I feel I can breathe easily for the first time in a long time. What I do notice is that I still have that knotted 'cancerous' sensation in my stomach. It's not as tense as before this session. A great weight on my shoulders has eased up, although something is still there and weighing me down slightly. My mind is clear, I can see what I have to achieve today, and it's progressing well.

Regarding the connection to the Universe, I notice it is still there, and it feels almost as strong as during my Sweet Spot experience yesterday. No, I don't think I'm going to turn into a new-age hippy or some spiritual guru. Yet I do believe that I have the potential to change into the person I was born to be. Better late than never, as the old saying goes.

Regarding my Mum, the most essential part for me is that I have released all that guilt and shame as I was feeling her presence surround me. It was her wish for me to be free from all that punishment and torture I have put myself under all these years. I willingly accept her offer as this release is something I desperately need. My love, admiration and respect for my Mum are as large and buoyant as they always were, and she has given me the sensation that I am freer and open to the world around me.

One Month Later...
I don't think my clarity of thought has ever been this good. I regularly see my past life thoughts flying around me, and much of the lifelong fog has lifted. Being around people is also

somewhat different; I am more relaxed in their company and can behave more naturally. Occasionally, I still feel unsure of what to say or do, yet I am more aware of how to think more relaxedly and approach some situations differently. This new openness in me is an excellent step in the right direction.

I love playing chess, although I don't get to play as often as I would like. Since experiencing this Sweet Spot, which is followed by the micro-dosing routine, I've noticed that my game has improved immensely. I am winning more often against the same opponents I regularly play. I can see the board clearly and how the pieces relate to each other.

Since completing this Sweet Spot experiment, I have not had one Dark Thought. My dreams are more interesting and 'fun'. I've had a few weird ones I haven't understood, but we'll put that down to having too much food and wine on the odd occasion.

Eating is still a bit of a mish-mash. For several days, I had reasonable control over my diet. Then my wife and I went to Prague for a short holiday, and I regressed. What chance did I have against all those delicious dumplings, traditional Czech food, and beer? Since coming back, I haven't noticed any improvement in my eating habits and have poor control over my diet again. Unfortunately, there is still a way to go on this one.

I have noticed that I am ageing physically since around the age of forty-eight, and a slight stiffness creeps in here and there. Maybe that's also linked to my poor diet and lack of fitness. However, since using psilocybin, some of the aches and pains have reduced. My leg still gives me jip, yet even that seems a little less severe than before.

Repeating an old cliché is like lifting a massive weight off my shoulders. Once those restrictive bonds have been broken, it can suddenly feel like an entirely different world exists before us, and it's not as bad as we make it out to be. For someone who hasn't experienced this, it may be very hard or impossible to understand what I mean by this. Now my shoulders feel lighter and I stand taller.

What a release.

I planned to stop this experiment here, but felt compelled to take it further and conduct another Sweet Spot session...

Schizophrenia and Micro-Dosing

Good moods are as fragile as eggs... and bad moods are as delicate as bricks.

David Mitchell

Regarding schizophrenia, I found this subject the most confusing of all the information out there when it comes to the use of psychedelics. It was when I accidentally stumbled across Robert Whitaker's brutally honest book, *Mad in America,* on the terrors that the mad and schizophrenic people have had to endure over the last several hundred years within institutions that I began to understand why.

This book highlights that medical treatment has focused more on hiding symptoms than finding a solution, thus hindering progress rather than advancing it. Although some things have changed for the better, this attitude continues even today.

I highly recommend reading this book if you have family or friends in a psychiatric ward or if you are visiting or planning to visit a psychiatrist, or even if you are considering entering a psychiatric hospital for treatment yourself, as it may help to give you a perspective on what might happen once you are, or someone else is, committed.

If you are already on medication, please read his other book, Anatomy of an Epidemic. This book explains how the different types of medication work, which theories and prescription medications are outdated and no longer considered relevant, and how to spot whether your doctor has kept up-to-date with the latest medical trends.

One surprising point that came across in this book concerns modern psychiatric treatment for people with schizophrenia. If they are treated in a developed country, then the chance of living a 'normal' life after starting medication and therapy is significantly less than 30%. Whereas those who live in a third-world, or in a country where medicine isn't as freely available, and receive only loving care and attention, have a greater than 70% chance of leading an everyday life again, e.g., getting married and going (back) to work a year or so later.

A second point which came out from this book is that those who are given medication tend to suffer more brain tissue loss of the frontal lobes, thus leading to cognitive impairment and worsening of the symptoms in general. There is also a tendency for these patients to die younger, having faced various complications like cardiovascular ailments, respiratory problems, metabolic illnesses, diabetes, kidney failure, etc. Not only that, but the severity of these conditions seems related to the amount of medication taken.

If one looks back at the history of the treatment of people with schizophrenia, there have been several highly successful and innovative solutions that do not involve medications at all. The first was the opening in 1796 of the William Tuke Retreat, named after its Quaker founder. This establishment still operates as an independent psychiatric hospital on the outskirts of York, UK, and is a registered charity.

These 'mad' people, in great contrast to the treatment of patients and the appalling conditions found in the Victorian 'mad houses', were considered intelligent and were treated with respect. They had access to lovely accommodation, good food, and activities that included, for example, occupational therapy, handicrafts, reading, and writing. And not once in their time at this retreat was a doctor present to discuss or review their mental illness. In all, more than 70% were released within two years of admission, with very few returning after some form of relapse.

Another more recent example was the 'Soteria Research Project' founded by psychiatrist Loren Mosher in San Diego,

California, USA in 1971. This experiment was based on patients' feedback in various respite centres, which showed that what they wanted most was love, care and understanding rather than medication. From the start, it was clear that this shift, by focusing on their emotions for their treatment, was hugely beneficial. Patients quickly alleviated symptoms, had a healthier outlook on life, integrated better socially, and were less susceptible to relapses.

The problem for Mosher was that the NIMH (National Institute for Mental Health), which provided the funding for the programme, and the academics who sat on the NIMH grant-review committees were strongly influenced by the pharmaceutical industry. This influence led the NIMH committee to change the protocols to try to show that medication was more effective than love, care, and attention.

Unfortunately for Mosher, his unwillingness to follow these new protocols led him to be excluded from the project team entirely, despite the proven benefits of his method. Once his replacement took over, the new protocols were implemented, medication was given, and the focus on emotional therapy was stopped completely. This change eventually led to the project being scrapped altogether.

Regarding micro-dosing, there are several people out there who use psychedelics to help them along with their daily schizophrenic battles. Most of those who micro-dose or take more substantial doses tend not to be on medication. A problem for some who have schizophrenia is that once they come off medication, the symptoms can become worse than those they had before they even started their medication.

Schizophrenia is still not very well understood, even after all these years. Fortunately, experiments are currently being carried out with specialists at MAPS, such that the results are showing that LSD can help people with schizophrenia get their lives back on track quickly and effectively. So, the potential seems to be out there as an alternative.

Note: If you are diagnosed as schizophrenic, taking medication and are considering psychedelics, please speak with a specialist first to check whether the psychedelic you wish to take could interact negatively with your medication. Also, if you are already on medication, please don't just stop it, as that will probably mess you up more than you were before you started taking it. If you do wish to come off your medication, please speak to your doctor who prescribed it to you. If they recommended how to take it, then they should be able to advise you how to come off it without the risk of a significant relapse.

Sweet Spot No 2 – Detachment, Acceptance and Responsibility

Anxiety is the dizziness of freedom.

                              Søren Kierkegaard

I am taking this second Sweet Spot because of a significant issue that remains within me: my eating issue. Since completing the first Sweet Spot, I have put on a little more weight, which tells me that something is still blocking me and that I need to deal with it, so this is the subject for this session.

I planned this therapeutic session for the morning because the first Sweet Spot left me so energised and motivated that I thought it would be a good idea to make the most of the remaining time after the session. Let's run through the day's events, and I'll discuss what I have gone through.

I take my 3.6g dose with scrambled eggs while still half asleep. Eating is tough as I'm building up a taste aversion to them, so I have to force down the last few mouthfuls. Directly after that, I totter off to bed with a growling stomach and no morning coffee.

When it starts to kick in, my first experience is an intense burst of static in my head, a bit like what I could call very loud tinnitus or similar to a guitar cable jack plugged into the amplifier socket while it's still powered up. That noise rattles deep in my left ear, with some sound in my right.

The volume is so loud it drowns out all other external noises around me and makes me instinctively flinch. This noise lasts for a few seconds and then goes away. A few minutes later, it happens again. It feels and sounds as if it is rattling from one ear to the other through the lower part of the brain. This is fantastic because it is the first time I can consciously recall that my right ear has functioned in some way. As for the deeper meaning, I still have no idea. After testing my hearing several hours later, I'm still deaf as a post in my right ear, so nothing has changed here.

As the psilocybin continues to kick in, various forms and shapes fly by, linked with red. The bedsheets are wine red, as are the closed curtains. What is weird is that I am looking in from the outside of this experience. Although I am going through this, I am not a part of it, which annoys me. I try to get into the experience, but I can't. As my anger mounts, a part of me is telling me that I can't get angry when in a therapy session and that I should remain calm.

I try to focus on my key concern regarding diet, but because I am not a part of the trip, I try to step into it, but I am thrown back out again. It's as though all these great experiences are happening without me, and I can't participate in them or learn from them. Grr! I so want to get something from this today.

Then I see an old, withered man and an old, wrinkled woman within the experience as I am still outside it. They are both me. It hurts to stare, but my eyes are locked onto them. What I see bothers me, and I don't know what to think about it as I continue to watch them just sitting there, staring into space. I ask myself what this means, but no answers come forth. After a short while, they disappear, and at the same time, a question pops up from nowhere: Do I still have something to give to this life, or is my time up?

Simply put, this scares me, and I have difficulty dealing with it. I spiral down into some sadness and loneliness during this session when I consider that there is no answer to this question. By seeing myself as an old man and woman, have I given up on life? I need a new focus, but I still don't know what it should be. Maybe this is my way of telling myself that I will reach a grand old age and have plenty of opportunities before me? I hope so!

I now feel old, really old, within myself. I take the opportunity to say, 'This is the end, and my old life is over.'

Now what?' I don't realise it at the time, but later I recognise this as a kind of experience that death is okay and that it is simply the end of one phase and the start of the next. Reflecting on this point further, I notice for the first time that I am now ready to look death in the eye and that I can now confidently leave this physical world when the time comes to go back to my celestial home and that I have nothing to be afraid of at all.

After a while, I ask myself what I have to live for. I realise I have my beautiful and caring wife; she's everything I have and is important to me. I've never been reflective or philosophical about life or my past experiences. However, since my first Sweet Spot session, I have dug deeper into my thoughts and history.

I've never kept a diary of events, nor was I interested in doing so. Yet here, I find writing all this down excellent since it helps me reflect on what has happened and gain a deeper understanding of my experiences and life.

My original quest was to find what was blocking me with my eating and fitness habits, work through this, and remove the blockage(s) so that I could start eating normally and taking better care of my physical fitness. In this reflective phase, I begin to assess further what I have gone through over the years.

This experience shows me how alone I have been and how I am plagued by the frustrating feeling of wanting to be an active part of life and society, yet never actually being so. My current experience is merely highlighting my frustration.

I was conceived by accident and born out of wedlock in the late 1960s. In those days, it was a big thing, and pregnant mothers were not supported as they are today. Unfortunately, Mum was ignored by her boyfriend (my father) and was rejected by her father when she found out she was pregnant. Mum had to leave the family home to live with an aunt at the other end of the country.

One of her central dilemmas while carrying me was not knowing what to do; whether to keep me or to hand me over for adoption. That must have been not easy and soul-destroying for her. So, from day one of the realisation that I existed, I was, in a sense, already an outsider.

I don't blame Mum for what happened or for the heart-wrenching decisions she had to make. It must have been trying for her to be torn between such impossible choices, thrown out of the family home, and not having the support of the man who fathered me next to her.

At this point, Mum still did not know about his brutal side. The turmoil that Mum went through must have been horrendous for her, and I often think about how she had to carry those mental scars with her for the rest of her adult life.

From the instant of being born, I was put up for adoption. Mum returned a couple of days later for me before the adoption process was complete. I am eternally grateful to her for coming back. That was the first time I had been held in her (or anybody's) arms, and then I felt her undying love. As we were adjusting to a new life with each other in Salisbury, prospects looked much rosier for both of us.

That was until Mum's father decided to 'do the right thing'. He found my father and pressured him into marrying his daughter and taking full responsibility for her and his child. Please let's remember: It was nearing the end of the 1960s, and those generations that had gone through the war were dealing with their mental battle scars as well as coping with rationing and rebuilding a nation.

The attitudes were different then; they didn't have half the resources and options we have today. They did what they thought was best at the time concerning their education, beliefs, understanding and expectancies according to what they had been brought up to believe. It is only in this light that, considering what had happened, we can begin to imagine what they were going through, even if some of their decisions may seem strange today.

For the next seven years, both my mother and I had to endure constant physical and verbal abuse from my father. And as I grew, I also had to cope with my leg issues and being deaf in one ear. These challenges set me apart from other schoolchildren and increased my sense of isolation. And this is when I started comfort eating. As I grew older, I gradually forgot the original reason for my need for comfort food and would persuade myself when binge-eating that I enjoyed my food. I still eat a lot. Inside me, I still feel alone. And it's now clear what drove me to food and overeating of the wrong things.

Ten hours have passed, and I am still being hit with some psilocybin mini waves. I must piece together what happened and what to do next in those reflective moments. I now know I can die in peace, and I have no fear of death anymore. I now know I have a lot to give, but I don't know what, if that makes sense.

I now understand the cause of my eating issue, and I no longer feel lonely. If this is the case, then perhaps I should be able to start eating normally. The next few weeks will tell. However, I have a feeling it won't change.

So, has everything been uncovered and understood about this session? I don't think so. I guess there are still some open questions. Maybe I still need time to consider this further over the next few days.

I had hoped I could have made a connection with the Universe on this trip. But how could this have been possible if I had never been part of it? I was outside of it the whole time, and there wasn't any chance to enter it. I never met my Gatekeeper. It never felt right, nor did I feel prepared to have the right mental attitude. So, there is no connection to the Universe today.

On a more cheerful note, my wife had accidentally dropped a multi-coloured rope belt on the floor early in the morning before going to work. A couple of hours into the session, I needed a quick pit-stop and popped to the loo when the belt came to life.

It looked like a glistening multi-coloured spider/winged insect thing that danced on delicate legs as it continuously observed me. At first, I was in awe that something as large and beautiful as that was living in the bedroom, and then I grew curious as I had never seen such a colourful creature like that before, as I cautiously made my way around to inspect it. Once I realised it was harmless, I left it alone, as I didn't want to scare it. So, I hobbled over the rolling floor towards a series of dancing doors that barred my way to the loo and left it in peace.

The end of this session wasn't clear, and it didn't answer my questions or give me what I was looking for. This was the first time they hadn't responded to a question. Maybe the question was wrong, or this wasn't the right approach to this problem.

Six Days Later...

I've decided to take a 1g dose to focus on tidying up my loose ends regarding my dietary challenges in the hope of putting them behind me. I am hoping to be able to address any further mental issues that might still be flying around, as I don't believe I covered everything in my last sitting. This is how it goes...

After taking my 1000mg dose, I dutifully lie down in bed. Before the psilocin kicks in, I think about what I want to focus on: improving my diet, identifying the underlying issue, and implementing the right solution.

Within about fifteen minutes, I notice a light relaxedness come over me. It differs from the other times I have taken a light dose, as my head doesn't swim as much as usual. After a short while, I am within the experience, unlike the last time. As I go deeper and deeper into this trance-like state, I ask myself if I am ready to complete the previous stage of this part of the journey.

The answer I receive is 'yes', I am. Still, in this early part of the trance, I enter myself at a cellular level and find myself communicating with each cell to reprogramme them to their original function. This part lasts for about an hour.

The point arrives when I think it is time to get up, shower, and get on with the day. I stand up and notice a light, swimming sensation in the room, but that's fine as it isn't intense enough to bother me. When I go into our bright white bathroom, I notice I need to lie down again, which I do.

Next, I will meet some people from my past, mainly from my university days, or at least, the background scenery is near my old college. None of the people I meet are in contact with me now, and I have no real yearning to meet them again. All the people I met played a minor role in my life at the time. Nothing special happens; we talk to each other about various interesting subjects, and then they disappear.

Then the next interesting person comes along, and so on. After a while, I had had enough of meeting these people. Only after reflection a day later did it dawn on me what this part told me; these people represented potentially good friendships I had missed out on due to my belief that I didn't deserve them to be a part of my life.

Back to my trance state. I need to get back to the problem at hand. But no matter how hard I try, I can't seem to re-enter the problem. I see colours and shapes that drift around, and that's it. After a couple of hours, I get up frustrated with this 'irrelevant' experience I am having and head for the shower. The shower is good and refreshing, and washing the previous night's sleep out of me is wonderful.

Afterwards, I noticed I needed to lie down again and jump on the couch as I was now alone. I lay on the sofa and I enter into a deep trance.

This time, I met up with several of my previous girlfriends with whom I had ended the relationship. And although it was great to see and talk to them again, they looked just like they did the last time I saw them in real life. I started to assess each relationship and why I had ended it. I don't consider what we could have done differently in the relationship, but for some reason, I am justifying to myself why I ended the relationship with each of them. As I am going through my original reasons, something niggles me, as if to say that these weren't the real reasons that I had ended the relationships. In their defence, it wasn't because they had done or said something wrong or that there were any issues between us, which I have always known, but never thought much more about over the years.

Slowly, it became clear that each of those relationships was ready to move forward, and I couldn't cope with the responsibility of doing this. This revelation is telling me I was scared of committing myself to them.

Instead, I found different reasons to finish the relationships. I was running away from taking proper responsibility for these lovely, funny and caring women. I am only beginning to realise how much anguish and pain I have caused. My psychedelic experience today shows me that I was also running away from myself by re-creating a secure situation where I was alone again and couldn't potentially be hurt by anyone.

Not that anyone ever really did that to me, except for the one person I should have been able to rely on: my father. This revelation is a shock when that sudden 'aha' moment of understanding flashes before me.

In a trance, I have a flashback of once coming home around nine in the morning after a night out on the town. My mother was at her wits' end since she didn't know where I was. In those days, we didn't have mobile phones, and in the UK, nightclubs closed at two in the morning, so coming home no later than three in the morning was usually the norm.

Because of the unusual time I came home, she had thought, like all good mothers do, that something had happened to me. I now realise how much of a prat I had been (nicely put) as she needed to go to a hospital that day for an operation, and this added stress was too much for her. What hits me today is that I hadn't taken on any responsibility for my family. I now know that mentally I couldn't cope with what was happening to my key role model (mum) in my life, and it was easier for me to blank it out and not be there. This session brings home to me just how much anguish I had put Mum through that day.

This recognition of my lack of responsibility for others throughout my life has hit me hard. Upon reflection, continually feeding crap food into myself and abusing myself in one way or another is a form of self-punishment.

I am showing a lack of respect and responsibility towards myself. If I consider how I participate in fitness and sport, I do it for a short while, and then when I start making progress, I hinder my progress enough to ensure that I make no further improvements. The story of my life is now as clear to me as a hard slap across the face. I now know what the word 'responsibility' really means.

And now that I understand what happened in the past, I ended these relationships due to my fear of being there for these people and being responsible for them. That is linked with my impulse to make self-destructive decisions, and it shakes me to the core.

I discussed this with my wife later in the day, and she asked me a brilliant question: 'Now that you know you need to take more responsibility for your life, what do you need to do differently to achieve this, and how will you know when you have achieved it?'

I am overcome with a sensation of blank incomprehension. I stand motionless in the kitchen while holding a cup of tea with absolutely nothing on my mind. I decided to take a long walk and consider the first part of the question about taking responsibility for my life. I now know there are certain areas I need to take more control over, and this requires a conscious effort from my side.

So, going back to my original question, I have found out what causes me to overeat and why I gorge on particularly unhealthy things. The reasons are twofold.

First, I have always felt alone and could never be a part of the crowd, which has frustrated me immensely. To ease that frustration, I turned to food for comfort. The second is that due to being a loner and living with low self-esteem, I had overstepped my inner self-worth marker as soon as I felt I had achieved some success in life. And hence the vicious circle of eating junk food, doing inconsistent sport, distancing myself from my friends, ending my relationships, messing up my job, family, home, etc. What an idiot I've been all these years.

The Next morning

Although I didn't sleep much through the night, my brain worked ten to the dozen. When I finally fell asleep, I remembered one dream I had. That was of a new me who is fit, healthy, confident, and making a success of my life, while strengthening my social bonds with the people around me.

Yet, a small chain around me still holds me back. It gives me some hope that there is something more that I have to live for, even though I haven't freed myself completely. I feel good and am more self-motivated to break that last bond. Who wouldn't be after such a dream? Now let's see how life pans out and what I can do to encourage it...

Possible Reasons to Legalise or Decriminalise Psychedelics

As a retired physician, I can honestly say that unless you are in a serious accident, your best chance of living to a ripe old age is to avoid doctors and hospitals and learn nutrition, herbal medicine and other forms of natural medicine unless you are fortunate enough to have a naturopathic physician available. Almost all drugs are toxic and are designed only to treat symptoms and not to cure anyone.

Dr Alan Greenberg, MD

After completing these experiments and researching quite intensively, it becomes apparent that there is a lot of potential for more significant health benefits for both mental and physical issues from using psychedelics. Here I would like to consider a potential future and what options we have in front of us, as well as in some countries where they have already made progress with outstanding results, which gives greater hope that governments worldwide could follow in their footsteps.

We've seen, partly due to the significant research from David Nutt, that psychedelics are not as harmful as other legal and illegal drugs on the market, including prescription medication, tobacco, alcohol and opiates. Most of these particular drugs kill and maim more people than all of psychedelics put together.

Not only that, but psychedelics mainly trigger a serotonin release in comparison to the release of noradrenaline and dopamine. Amphetamines and opiates trigger significantly higher levels of noradrenaline and dopamine release that can lead to possible addiction. We've also discussed that psychedelics could be used to help fight against PTSD, cancer, fear of death, pain, neurological illnesses, and help solve relationship issues and family disputes. We've also mentioned that in contrast to the adverse social effects of alcohol, psychedelics can help to reduce neighbourhood violence and to promote community relationships.

When we consider why the majority of world governments ignore the fact that the use of psychedelics could give them the potential to provide a helpful service to the people they are meant to represent?

Could it be that politicians are scared of finally admitting the truth and have made a massive mistake all these years? Could it be that it is more convenient for governments to ignore the facts by spreading untruthful propaganda to make their job in office easier?

Could it be that the Pharma industries are scared of losing out on sales and profits for some of their products, which psychedelics may immediately replace, by funding our politicians to allow more dangerous drugs to flood the market, and at the same time to keep the safe and effective ones banned? Could governments have no interest in returning the trust and respect the electorate has given them?

Could it be that the politicians fear losing their power and influence as the primary motivating force behind this phoney drug war? Or could it be that governments see this anti-psychedelic propaganda as a valuable tool for deflecting from the other political mistakes which some are making? Or maybe it's a mix of them together.

And lastly, why do we, the people, just accept the adverse effects of alcohol and tobacco that maim and kill millions of our family and friends each year, which cost us vast sums of money?

As noted in Tom Wainwright's book: *Narconomics: How To Run A Drug Cartel*, in 1971, President Nixon said that 'Public enemy number one in the United States is drug abuse. To fight and defeat this enemy, it is necessary to wage a new, all-out offensive.' As a side-note, he also said in a private conversation that was recorded, "To take somebody that's smoked some of this stuff (cannabis), put him into jail with a bunch of hardened criminals... that's absurd... There must be different ways than jail." This book won't discuss why he did nothing to support that statement.

What we want to cover is Nixon's problem with drug-taking that didn't concern domestic consumption, but the use of drugs by US soldiers in Vietnam. It was this he wanted to hide from the public. At the time, about 67% of soldiers were using cannabis, and about 50% were using both cannabis and opiates, with a significant number of these soldiers showing some signs of addiction to other hard drugs, too.

Nixon feared that this drug use, which was an accepted means of dealing with battlefield issues, was fuelling the growing hippie and flower-power movement in the US. What Nixon ignored was that most of the soldiers effortlessly stopped using opiates on their return home. And if he had ceased the war on drugs at that point, maybe the issues wouldn't have grown to the exaggerated proportions we have today.

Nixon believed that by introducing idealistic legislation, he could show his concern for the health and welfare of humankind in achieving a 'drug-free world'. However, he meant illegal drugs only, regardless of how many people had died from legal ones. He maintained that (illegal) drug addiction was a grave evil with accompanying social and economic dangers for all of us.

And finally, Nixon pointed out that each American had a duty to prevent and combat this evil. I love how religion is constantly brought into politics to influence the way the average person thinks, especially when we consider that religions in their early days appear to be one of the most significant users of psychedelics. This moralistic approach by Nixon, accompanied by an uneducated propaganda campaign, set the standard path for the rest of the world to follow unthinkingly.

The only problem is that this war on drugs has cost governments around the world billions and billions of wasted pounds and dollars, especially when we consider that Illegal drug sales account for the second largest trade volume in the global economy after oil. Yet, these not-so-harmful and unlawful drug sales are worth more than £300 billion per year to the global economy.

This figure is equivalent to about 1% of total trade worldwide. Imagine what each respective government could do for its citizens with a proportional slice of this very expensive pie instead of just throwing this potential income down the proverbial drain if these drugs were made legal.

Those Losing Out

The question I hear you asking is, 'Surely all this money spent fighting against drugs has reduced the demand, hasn't it? Well, not exactly. According to David Nutt in his book *Drugs Without The Hot Air,* over the period 1998 to 2008, opiate sales increased from nearly 13 million kilograms to more than 17 million kilograms; cocaine from just over 13 million kilograms to around 17 million kilograms and cannabis from about 110 million kilograms to 160 million kilograms.

It's a continually growing multi-billion-dollar industry for the mafia and other drug cartels. They then freely launder their money through our banking systems with the support of a few corrupt politicians and businesses. Unfortunately, almost none of this money earned from the sale of illegal drugs finds its way back into improving our domestic market or towards services for those who need help the most.

One of the most frequently employed arguments used by the government is to justify the banning of cannabis and psychedelics on the ground that they are a gateway toward harder drugs. As previously discussed, this is mostly a dishonest debate, since we now know that by far the biggest 'gateway drug' is alcohol. Not only that, if someone is predestined to use hard drugs, they will eventually get there regardless of what they first start with, and it is these people who need the help the most. Yet psychedelics, in contrast, can provide us with one of the safest and most effective therapies against addiction.

There is, however, another and more insidious gateway to the taking of harder drugs, and that is through our prison system for those incarcerated. In the UK, around 20% of prisoners are addicted to opiates. Many of those are inmates who try heroin for the first time. By illegalising drugs such as cannabis and other psychedelics, the government is contributing to this problem by increasing prison numbers by focusing on the small-time users at the very bottom of the drug chain.

It is these people who have handled small quantities of psychedelic drugs, as well as those who use them for personal consumption only. Many of the larger dealers and cartel bosses, even if they are caught, can usually afford to pay for expensive lawyers. These lawyers, in turn, can often organise a quick-release programme for their well-connected clients.

Thus, by targeting the small fry, the government can only scratch the surface at the wrong end of the industry chain. Anyone who has seen the brilliant TV series, *The Wire*, or *Breaking Bad* will know what I mean. It's worth mentioning another critical TV series, called *Oz*. It shows the problems within our prisons when small-time users are treated the same as and kept with hardened and dangerous criminals, thus leading more innocent people into crime or an early death.

Continuing on the theme of gateway to harder drugs, Tom Wainwright in his eye-opening book, *Narconomics: How To Run A Drug Cartel*, mentions that there is a new lethal gateway to opioid addiction, and that is through our doctors, the general practitioner (GP). Doctors often prescribe heroin-based painkillers for patients, and it is these prescriptions that are renewed often enough to allow addiction to get a foothold.

Once the GP stops providing a new prescription, their patients' problems begin.

Buying this same medication on the black market is too expensive for most people, so they start to purchase heroin directly from the drug dealer because it is ultimately much cheaper and more readily available. Recently, there has also been a demographic change in opiate usage and addiction. In the early years of its popularity, men and fewer younger women were initially the main users. Today, however, this dominant group of addicts are white, affluent and older women.

Another related issue causing social unrest concerns the often and rather heavy-handed police actions, mostly in socially deprived areas of our major cities, which are conducted at a ratio of about 7:1 against non-whites. These include arbitrary 'stop-and-search' actions that can efficiently fuel racial tensions and help incite street riots, as we have previously seen several times in various countries around the world. The UK and the US are excellent examples of this.

On the other side of the coin, many terminally ill patients die in discomfort due to a lack of appropriate painkillers. The use of morphine is highly regulated worldwide, and this may help with the pain, but it prevents suffering patients from gaining the mental relief they need.

As we have seen, cannabis seems to be a highly effective remedy against pain, as are other psychedelics, such as LSD, mescaline and psilocybin, which can also reduce the fear of death and allow for a smoother transition out of this world. Each of us should be able to decide how we die rather than have it dictated to us by the government.

For me, one of the other unnecessarily restrictive aspects endorsed by governments is that once a drug becomes illegal at its highest category, research is practically forbidden. This research could and should be happening to benefit everybody's mental health. For example, by using psychedelics to alleviate addiction, pain, death, cognitive issues, neurological illnesses, etc, this would free the UK's NHS resources and save huge sums which are otherwise spent on procuring expensive medication, etc.

At the time of writing, the Institute for Economic Affairs in the UK has estimated that legalising cannabis alone would earn the UK treasury around £1 billion a year and save the NHS around £300 million annually. In the case of cannabis, it is said that legalisation would virtually eliminate black-market dealings. So, suppose it's suitable for the husband of a drug-opposing politician, MP Victoria Atkins, with the support of the Prime Minister, Theresa May, that enables her partner to earn large amounts of money from growing and selling cannabis. In that case, it must also be suitable for the general population, too.

On the other hand, there is Al Qaeda, who generate funding from the sale of opium and cannabis to purchase weapons for their wars. Sadly, these weapons are sold legally by our government-supported manufacturers. Maybe with all that money flowing into their pockets, the governments do have some reason to agree on the war on drugs after all! Hmm, composure, Neil.

Now, where was I? Ah, yes, well, at least a good chunk of these mafia, terrorism and blood money issues would disappear practically overnight once psychedelics (and harder drugs) were made legal.

There is another concern that needs to be considered, and that relates to the drug users themselves. In the UK, around 85% of shoplifting and 80% of burglaries are carried out by approximately 300,000 heavy drug users. There are approximately 30,000 of these users responsible for about half the brutal drug-related crimes that happen.

Naturally, this is another significant cost to the taxpayer, costing around £11 billion yearly. It surely makes more sense to have psychedelic drugs legalised/decriminalised so that all users can be supported in their most difficult moments in life. Canada, Portugal, the Netherlands and South Africa are the best examples of countries giving this support to hard drug users, which would provide the taxpayer with a proper share of that wasted tax money back in our pockets.

Making Comparisons

Now let's consider a perspective from the eyes of a politician by comparing legal and illegal drugs. According to David Nutt, this is something that the MP, Jacqui Smith, is wholly opposed to doing. Worldwide, tobacco alone has an impressive kill of around 5 million people yearly, and alcohol has a modest kill of approximately 1.5 million people each year. That's 6.1 million people who die from these two legal drugs yearly.

In comparison, psychedelic drugs kill about 200,000 people worldwide annually. That's nearly 31 times more deaths from just tobacco and alcohol in comparison to the death count from all psychedelics grouped. Based on this, I now understand why politicians don't want these figures compared with each other, because it would be another reason to throw out their senseless anti-drug campaign onto their ever-growing scrapheap of bad political decisions.

If governments were to admit these statistical truisms, it might become somewhat more challenging for them to demand further funding from the general citizen to fund the war on drugs. Not only that, the cheaper option, namely the use of psychedelics would contribute positively to the treatment of PTSD sufferers, addicts, anorexics, depressives, asthmatics, cancer patients, diabetes, epileptics, paraplegics, schizophrenics and those suffering from Alzheimer's, arthritis, autism, cystic fibrosis, glaucoma, Huntington's, insomnia, migraines and cluster headaches, hepatitis, multiple sclerosis, muscular dystrophy, osteoporosis, rheumatism, stress disorders, Tourette's and others. I have included a more extensive list near the end of the book for those who wish to investigate this further.

And if I'm wrong, then what return does the government have to show for this unrelenting war against illegal drugs that is supposedly conducted in the name of its citizens?

I've mentioned before that the trade in psychedelics is worth around £300+ billion per year. But how much does it cost our citizens to fund this war on drugs? Worldwide, we have unwittingly contributed more than $2.5+ trillion to the war against drugs over the last 50 years.

What is worse is that it has only brought us a massive financial loss, unnecessary deaths and a rapidly diminished quality of life. As a taxpayer and a person who is at risk of some illness that psychedelics could help me with, I find this approach from our politicians absurdly expensive and irresponsible.

Thankfully, the political tide is slowly changing. Several retired politicians have commented that legislation needs to change, and I wholeheartedly agree. Shame these same UK politicians didn't have the spine when they were in office to fight for it and implement their recommended changes instead of leaving it to the leaders of more forward-thinking countries.

We even had one of our ex-Prime Ministers, David Cameron, say that we should be tough on drugs. However, his punishment when he was caught with cannabis in his younger years was to be given lines. This type of punishment involves writing the exact phrase repeatedly, as Bart Simpson does on the classroom board in the opening credits of *The Simpsons*.

Yeah, I know, it was a challenging and gruelling punishment for Cameron, and I suppose his stance against cannabis and other psychedelics is related to this horrific treatment he had inflicted on him. He was lucky to come from a rich, privileged and influential family. But had he been poor or non-white, however, he would probably have been imprisoned for a long time with no prospect of a proper career thereafter, even with the small amount he had on him.

Finally, if this expensive and fruitless war on drugs has had no effect whatsoever over the last fifty years, isn't it now time to change our incorrect perceptions of psychedelics for future generations?

A Possible Future...

Some attitudes are changing, and other countries are leading the way. In Canada, Portugal, Spain, the Netherlands, South America and South Africa and maybe more as this book goes to print, medical and recreational cannabis is now legalised/decriminalised. In the UK, some police forces are already looking the other way when people are found carrying small amounts of cannabis or when a few plants are grown at home for private use.

However, legal proceedings still follow once it becomes apparent that the quantity produced is 'too much' for personal consumption. These are all steps in the right direction. But what else can be done?

One option would be to sell psychedelics from dedicated shops in a similar way to how cannabis is sold in the Netherlands. These shops are licensed, and cannabis is freely used. A total ban on the sales of alcohol and the smoking of tobacco exists while visiting such premises.

This freedom gives users the chance to enjoy their consumption without the fear of prosecution and the associated risks of tobacco smoke and alcohol. Interestingly, however, once a tourist leaves the centre of Amsterdam, the touristic coffee shops are hard, if not impossible, to find. Why? The residents know how to get along with cannabis, which is generally accepted and casually smoked everywhere.

Another simple option would be to have recreational shops that sold such psychedelics and related paraphernalia in one place. Licensing would help ensure the quality of the drugs, allowing people to relax and not be under the constant threat of police raids. A great benefit here would be the creation of a new breed of consumer specialists who could give the proper advice when needed.

Even if this is too much for each country's government to accept at this time, at least pharmacies could be licensed to start selling psychedelics instead. What matters, especially in the early stages of setting these systems up, is that the product source is consistent, trustworthy and reliable.

A further step forward could be to have certain psychedelic café shops with membership access only, where the consumption and health of members can be monitored, along with a support network available for those who need it. Spain has taken this idea one step further to include harder drugs, too. This idea might sound extreme.

However, there have already been demonstrable benefits concerning quality control of the drugs themselves, the availability of clean and new syringes, and the provision of medical assistance and professional support for addicts. The number of addicts and new cases of transmissible diseases such as HIV and hepatitis have dropped, and fewer families have been separated from their loved ones by not sending them to prison.

In Liverpool, Dr John Marks set up a treatment programme in 1982 that helped addicts obtain a regular supply of clean needles as well as free prescription heroin, cocaine and crack cocaine. They were then able to take their drug of choice in a safe environment, as well as receive specialist advice on how best to come off their drug.

A couple of the reasons for the success of this project were that users felt safe and secure in a relaxing environment. Whereas in complex, cold and artificial clinical settings or with the risk of arrest or attack, etc, the patients had significantly more 'bad' and unnerving experiences, such that the results were not as beneficial for the user's drug withdrawal.

As this programme got underway, the police reported in their end-of-year statistical report that there had been a 94% drop in theft, robberies and property crime and a reduction in drug use. Another benefit was that more users in the treatment centres remained HIV free (due to access to clean needles) and, at a later date, were able to return to work and become a part of society again. That was until the US government (Bill Clinton) in 1995 forced the UK (John Major) to stop this project, which the British government did without question.

One of the positive knock-on effects of decriminalising cannabis in the Netherlands is that it now has one of the lowest levels of heroin abuse in Europe. This is because those who are at a higher risk of addiction and wish to use cannabis never have to contact a dealer. Instead, they are in a safe environment and can obtain professional help in many mental and physical health areas.

Another example is Switzerland's heroin maintenance programme, which has operated for around twelve years. Over this period, the number of registered heroin users has fallen by 82%. The programme has helped addicts to deal with their substance abuse and to re-enter society.

The EU has even recognised the advantages of safe injection sites (for cocaine, heroin and crack cocaine), and these have been set up in over sixty cities. Here, users can safely take their drugs without fear of arrest.

One thing we tend to forget is that most of those who turn to drugs (legal and illegal) do so because they are struggling to deal with some problem. We all carry some baggage from our past, but I think we also need to be less critical and judgmental of those who are less able to cope with their problems than others. We should be facing and dealing with these problems, rather than trivialising them as many seem to do. The above points seem like a great way forward.

What if psychedelics were to be decriminalised, but not legalised? Instead of the police targeting the deprived social classes and those in difficulties looking for some escapism, they are unnecessarily over-filling prisons with these small-time users, and the police could start to focus on the bigger, bad boys. Also, fewer criminal records would be handed out to those who don't deserve them, thus protecting many people's futures.

Another knock-on effect is to allow more small-time psychedelic users back to work, allowing more legitimate money to flow through the financial system, from which we can all find some benefit. Perhaps governments could find themselves in a bit of a dilemma here. If all illegal mass growers and distributors were arrested (mafia, cartels, etc), who would supply the decriminalised market?

As seen with Leah Betts and many others, who have unfortunately died from misinformation on drugs, the government needs to promote safety among drug users. This support must include more on-the-spot access to crucial information and centres where drug users can obtain this from trained helpers, as discussed above.

Uninformed propaganda, such as that pushed out by the government during the 1980s and 1990s, needs to be replaced by verifiable and well-researched facts, as exemplified by David Nutt and other responsible scientists. Those who need help and advice can then be actively encouraged and provided with early and safe access to those drugs which have been proven to be the most helpful in their most difficult times. Sufferers should not be forced, as I am, to resort to illegal experimentation to get their life back.

The government should empower hospitals to treat those who have reacted badly to their use of psychedelics with experts to help, if necessary, as done for alcohol and other addictive legal substances. The current and long-standing argument is that hospitals won't have enough beds because it is too expensive for hospitals.

In the long term, however, the essential nuances to treat such people would be by the freed-up hospital beds in dealing with fewer victims due to excessive drinking, less street violence, less domestic abuse and a reduction of other violent crimes. This idea sounds like a win-win situation for everybody, doesn't it?

Portugal carried out something similar. Cocaine, heroin and cannabis are still illegal, but carrying small amounts is no longer punished. The drugs are confiscated, and the user goes in front of a discussion board for assessment to determine whether the user is addicted. After evaluation, they are warned, fined or referred for rehab as appropriate. So, how has Portugal benefited from this scheme?

Firstly, there was a significant drop in the number of those newly infected with HIV. In 2000, 1,430 new cases were reported when this scheme started. In 2008, there were only 352. This result alone is a fantastic drop in the number of newly infected drug users. In 1998, 23,500 heroin addicts were in treatment, whereas by 2010, ten years after this new system became operational, 40,000 had registered.

At first glance, these figures seem to show a negative trend, but the opposite is true. Many of the addicts knew they had a problem but were scared to come forward and ask for help before this change was implemented. For example, the risk of users landing in jail and subsequently losing their income and their family was just too great to ask for help. Once that risk was removed, it allowed more users to come forward, ultimately saving lives, families, jobs and freeing up the burden of overcrowded prisons.

Also, as a secondary knock-on effect, there is less peer pressure placed on youngsters to try such drugs in the first place. Here we are talking, of course, about harder drugs such as heroin and cocaine. The small-time, private users of cannabis are not affected by the majority of issues mentioned above – no HIV, no physical addiction and no families unnecessarily being ripped apart from its effects.

Fortunately, as I have said before, more and more people are starting to see through the hollowness and falseness of government propaganda in this phoney war on drugs, and if continued, can only lead to a further loss of trust in our political system, above all by our younger generations. I hope our governments start to choose a different strategy very shortly, and I hope they begin to protect those people who are more likely to experiment with drugs in the first place.

The big pharma industry is a cartel business, just like an auto or TV production company, that aims to win customers and earn more profits for itself and its shareholders. There's no doing good for the community. For them, the more medication that appears and is sold on the market, the better the turnover and profits, all with immunity. And who better than a doctor to market and push their products?

I understand that, as a business, the Pharma cartel needs their customers to think they need a different medication for different 'issues', regardless of the damage they could cause, rather than encouraging people to change their diet or lifestyle as a first step. I disagree with this.

Imagine what would happen if instead of focusing all its time and energy on supporting the Pharma industry, the politicians concentrated on representing the unfortunate people and families that have unnecessarily died or have become ill from wrong prescriptions, mis-information, reactions, etc, as well as by supporting those lives affected when essential drugs are withdrawn from the market.

Wouldn't it be great to end imposed Pharma companies when users suffer in some way, such that the money would be used to support their victims, just like it is in some other industries?

I'm back in Utopialand again, aren't I?

Don't get me wrong. Modern medicine has its place. However, I think it needs to be selective and used as a last option, not as the first and only option. For life-threatening situations, it has its rightful place in our society.

This discussion leads us to a final, but central theme in our conversation about the future of psychedelics. There is a need for active and unbiased research, unlike the underlying Ricaute report discussed earlier. One growing problem is that distrust in our governments has grown so large over the years that more and more ordinary people are not listening to their advice and feel obligated to experiment with psychedelics on their own.

And as I have often said, psychedelics seem to be an effective option in helping us deal with the myriad of mental and physical issues many millions are fighting against. It's a great shame the government has forced this potentially hugely valuable source of health care underground, making the internet and feedback from friends or acquaintances virtually the only sources of practical advice available.

Are not the lives of the citizens the government is meant to represent supposed to be more important than the profits made by pharmaceutical companies? Are we voting the right people into power to give us the proper support and protection we need? We need more people-focused politicians to speak out for our needs than we currently have.

Then there are those who, due to the government's unresearched propaganda, have lost years of their life because psychedelics have been banned. As I said earlier, I am one of those who once believed all the political bullshit flying around. In my youth, I trusted the government to make the right decisions for my welfare, but all their propaganda has turned out to be useless hot air, and I was just one of their political victims.

As I have said, I may be breaking the law, but I have my life back. For me, this is worth the risk of possible criminal prosecution. Yet many have been afraid to take this risk for whatever reason and have ended up killing themselves through depression or dying as a result of a Big Pharma drug overdose. Other unfortunate people have ended up in a hospital, ending up in some other institution or dying destitute on the streets. That is a regrettable state of affairs for those living under a political system meant to support and protect us.

We can only be thankful that more and more people are taking the initiative into their own hands and doing what they can to rescue their lives at the risk of prosecution. My hat goes off to them, and I can only thank them for taking the risk in publishing their findings and trying to reach out to fellow sufferers. Their feedback has helped me immensely. I hope that before my time is up, the laws will have changed enough to allow an open and free society (at least with psychedelics) once again.

If you wish to read further on how some of our international governments have enabled the drug mafia to thrive and make illegal drugs into a global mass money-making adventure, how the banks and politicians work hand in hand with criminals and on how we are unnecessarily fleeced from our taxes, please read *McMafia,* by Misha Glenny. Another great book on how drug cartels work and how the government has got things wrong and, in some cases, right, is Narconomics: How to Run A Drug Cartel, by Tom Wainwright.

Sweet Spot No 3 – Self-Discovery

Progress, not perfection.

Complex PTSD: From Surviving to Thinking, *Pete Walker*

Since my second Sweet Spot session, I thought I had some things in my life more under control, but upon reflection, I don't believe this is the case. I do notice differences, yet there is still a level of lethargy that hangs over me. It's much less than before, but it's still too much for my liking, and I need to do something about it.

I discuss this lethargy problem with my wife, and she thinks there is still something inside me that is holding me back. In a nutshell, I am still directionless and not as motivated due to some other issue I have remaining concerning dying, which I've had for a while. It's not the fear of death itself, which is the issue I had faced up to in my previous session.

It's more a fear that this could happen anytime soon, so what's the point of starting anything new? And it is this thought that provides the fuel to that lacklustre feeling inside me. If I try to locate this feeling of emptiness, it seems to be all around and within me. It's everywhere, whichever direction I turn, and this always remains with me.

My wife thinks it is linked to the last business I had grounded. There was a time in the early days when I thought it wouldn't survive and that I would have to close the shop permanently. Fortunately, that never happened, and I was able to build it up and sell it at the right time. Maybe she is right because my thoughts revolve around not wanting to go through those same challenges of starting a business again.

Not only that, if something goes wrong in a new venture and I lose the investment, then that's a good chunk of my life savings gone, and I'm not willing to risk that.

I believe the main reason for my lethargy has to do with the near-death experience I had when I was in hospital with blood sepsis and the related mental conflict I have between realising the difference between actual mortality and perceived immortality. I think this conflict is the challenge I have to face, and somehow, I need to replace my negative images of death with the realisation that I am healthy enough to live for a good few more years yet.

Now, it's down to business to see which of us is right. Where are those magical mushrooms of mine...?

Today, I give myself plenty of time to wake up. I have decided not to rush into it like I did the last time, and only start the session when I have had a cup of coffee. I measure out my 3.6g of dried ground mushrooms as my scrambled eggs gently cook nearby. I mix the two after turning off the heat. My nose turns up at the thought of that horrible psilocybin mushroom taste. Even their smell is bad enough to make me want to gag.

My setting is slightly different this time around. The curtains are open; it is a grey and rainy day outside. I think there's nothing worse than tripping inside on a sunny day, as I want to be outside in it. One aspect I have kept the same is that I have no music playing. I want to have no other external influences on what I am about to experience.

This is what happens...

It starts almost like the end of the book/film where Dorothy in *Wizard of Oz* repeats to herself 'There's no place like home,' until she is taken back home to her aunt's and uncle's house. In my case, I have the 'What's stopping me from getting on with my life?' mantra playing in my head. I faithfully keep this going even as I notice light-headedness that overtakes me.

This time, I don't have any whizzing patterns or colours flying around. Instead, this is a lot calmer, almost still, and everything in my inner mind is white. And in this calming whiteness, I go deeper into the experience, which begins with simple and casual discussions with nondescript people I don't know or remember from my life.

Out of frustration, just talking to these people, I started to search for what I needed to release from within, but none of the ideas I had before this trip came up. I continue to search for them in vain. Maybe I am searching for the wrong thing, I don't know. And if that's the case, what and how will I recognise it when it does appear?

And as the search goes on, the whiteness grows darker and the open space closes up. I reluctantly enter a dark, eerie corridor, so no light penetrates it. I don't want to go down this bleak, dark, neglected passage that is rank and stinks of putrid filth. I want to get out of there as quickly as possible. What could there be in such a horrible place which could help me?

Then, the tiniest ray of light catches a slight movement under a grubby old-fashioned industrial-type radiator. At first, I decided to ignore it. However, during the short time I have been carrying out these therapeutic trips, I have learnt one thing: nothing is superfluous in these visions. Maybe it has some meaning for me, so I bend and reach for it.

Carefully, I pick it up between my fingers and twist my hand around so that it lies gently in the palm of my hand. It is immediately apparent that I have found what I am looking for, which isn't what I expect to discover. In the palm of my hand, I am holding a tiny, withered, neglected, unloved foetus.

And that poor little thing is me.

This tiny thing curls away from me and indicates that it wants to go back under the radiator to wither away and die quietly. It doesn't feel loved, it doesn't feel wanted, and it doesn't think it has a place in this world. It just wants to return to the dark and protective womb again, where it can't be disturbed. But because there is no womb to crawl into, it is lying there, alone in the filth, merely waiting for that last sap of energy to leave its pathetic little body.

First, I hold him close, but the little me on my palm rejects my offer. I keep him warm and clean his grimy little body. Over time, the surroundings grow brighter as I see the baby getting stronger. Only his right leg remains withered. It is now up to me to give life and hope to this person, to show him how much I love him and that I have immense respect for him after what he has gone through. I must show him how he can grow in new situations, as his trust in me grows. Maybe I should rewrite that last part as 'my trust in me grows'.

As the baby begins its early childhood, I see myself as a little girl. She is wearing a summer dress, dancing, skipping around, and enjoying her freedom with two good legs. It is a weird sensation being someone else, especially not being a boy. As for experiencing two good legs for the first time, and I can move properly, this is indescribably fantastic.

This dual activity of being male and female gives me a fuller perspective. I now understand better how similar we are to each other and how much we need to rely on each other within our gender and life roles. As my younger version now reaches his teens, I experience being one of the lads and as part of a group. I am strong, reliable, funny, open, and appealing to the girls.

And standing next to this teen, I see myself as a wounded and sad transvestite who is hovering over a confused young man who is deep in thought. Each of these people I represent has different needs and has something special to give to others. Although I don't understand everything, I now realise that for most of my life I have remained oblivious to these facets of myself.

As these individual personalities grow and develop, this vicariously personified 'me' reaches his early twenties. I see myself as a black man with a shaved head who comes across as a trustworthy and reliable person, yet I experience the racial hatred and isolation from non-blacks that comes his way. It is neither a pleasant nor a justified experience. I interpret this as a symbolic representation of the issues that caused the bullying and torment inflicted on me as a child.

It doesn't matter who a person is, where they come from, or their background; we all have the same feelings, expectations, and needs. I realise how I need to stand up for myself and others. This feeling of tolerance towards others, regardless of race, was never my strong point. Those who know me well have known me as a person who took a rather blinkered and black-and-white approach to life and others.

As I look at the new me, I realise that I have been carrying this neglected self within me all my life. I recognise, too, that over the years I have nurtured this 'other' me, the one who is a withered and unwanted baby. I have, for all these years, encouraged this lonely person to go back into the womb and die. In a sense, I have become that womb within that has isolated me from outside contact.

It's my protection against being hurt again like I was as a child, and that served as a justification for my self-pity. That womb existed as my sanctuary, an isolation chamber of misery and (dis)comfort. It was intended to be where I wanted to have that last breath all alone, instead of it being a place of loving conception and growth, by providing the start of a new spiritual and physical beginning. Yet I am now ready to start to dismantle it, that 'cancer', that sits like a heavy weight in my stomach.

In my eagerness, I break the womb's walls down, and they collapse so that it can never be used again. And as that desolate womb crumbles into nothingness, he and I become one. I merge with this once neglected baby who has grown through many different personalities to be a strong and confident man filled with love, hope, aspiration, and respect for himself and others. This newborn me has so much to give and live for. It fills me with a desire to live fully and makes me feel whole again.

I sense a new strength and pride growing within myself. I have every reason to walk tall and be proud of my history, the battles I have lost and those I have surprisingly won. Despite a long journey ahead, I have every right to hold my head up high. The difference is, I can now see the road ahead a little clearer. Before, this road was enveloped in a thick fog, hiding the continuous violent storms raging around. I only realise how little fog I have removed over these past months.

I open my eyes and see myself in a new light. My hands are those of someone in their fifties, yet my mind is that of someone younger. I see the neglect, the abuse and the self-imposed suffering I have gone through. I now understand the drama I went through in my past. I feel a new, confident, and robust energy burning inside me.

There are no watertight plans, guarantees, or promises in life. Future challenges require overcoming a wide range of problems as part of life's rich experience. Once we choose to stop caring, giving, and receiving, our physical life is mostly at an end.

For the next hour, my mind continues to process what I have gone through to understand better what has happened. I will analyse this for several days, if not weeks or months. I do believe this is a significant discovery I have made today.

Unfortunately, I haven't been able to include everything I have experienced here, not because I don't want to tell you. So much happened at such an astonishing rate, and the changes were so powerful and profound that I cannot remember all the thoughts and events.

I noticed in this session that everything seemed real, with clarity, and focused. I participated and interacted personally the whole time, which is entirely different from my previous Sweet Spot session. Admittedly, doing the first Sweet Spot session, I could see things from my perspective, but it was visually very different from this one. This experience seemed to include every nerve and muscle fibre in my body.

This time, the room wasn't spinning, no weird colours were flying around, and no other interferences were happening. It was all minimalistic.

And when that little foetus lay in the palm of my hand, I felt its cold, shivering body penetrating deep into my skin, and I can still feel that coldness today. I felt the weak pulse of its little heart as it pulled away from me, wanting to leave me to curl up and die. That bothered me so much that this memory will remain with me for the rest of my life.

Two Weeks Later...

For two weeks now, my brain has been almost continually processing those experiences, and I have had several flashbacks and dreams. I can't remember what they were, but they were not Dark Thoughts. They were light and easy, and they gave me no stress. When I woke up each morning, I felt good and refreshed, my heart rate was light and steady, and I felt physically and mentally refreshed. I don't think I had ever dreamt in such a relaxed and natural manner as this before.

Then, at the end of these two weeks, I had a kind of Dark Thoughts dream. But there was a difference to it. In this darkness, I was shaking an old self from me, as one does with a long coat that sits heavily on the shoulders. It didn't leave me stressed as the other Dark Thoughts have done. My heart wasn't pounding like it usually does when I wake up from such nightmares. That morning, I got out of bed and restructured my diet. I hope this has a longer-term effect on my health...

One Month Later...

I still have some control over my eating, but it's a battle. I still have the occasional pang for something sweet, but after a few minutes, it passes. Overall, my weight has dropped 3.5kg. If I look at myself in the mirror, I look thinner, and my face looks healthier, too, compared to how I was just a short while ago. I have only another 16kg to lose before I reach my ideal weight... It's hard work, and I hope the effort is worthwhile.

Another change sport-wise is that I have been able to train a little more intensively, and I am enjoying the time I am investing in this. I am stronger and physically more aligned. This is an experience I've never really had before. The sport I am doing is relatively basic and not doing a great deal for my heart. It became clear one day when my wife and I had gone for a short walk. After walking up a relatively steep hill that was probably no more than about fifty metres high, my heart was pounding very fast and hard. This lack of fitness shocked me somewhat. I have to work on this.

Two Months Later...

It just gets better. I've had no Dark Thoughts at all. My dreams are light, I wake up more motivated and refreshed, and I get up earlier. It's wonderful. My writing is progressing well, yet I realise there is still room for more fine-tuning. My days are more structured than before, and I make more use of the time I have each day. It's not perfect, but it's heading in the right direction.

My thinking is clearer and more positive. Some negative thoughts slip in occasionally, but with some effort and control, I can hinder them somewhat and encourage myself to start thinking more optimistically again. Over time, these negative thoughts are happening less and less, but they aren't disappearing altogether.

My fitness has reached another level. I have increased my level of physical activity and am improving my heart's strength by participating in HIIT training. Given the imbalance within my legs, I have to be careful, as my left one tends to do most of the work. So, my heart and I are enjoying this new training regime. I notice that climbing the stairs has become easier, and I am not puffing as much when I reach the top of our apartment. My only concern is that the sport isn't flowing, and neither am I doing it as willingly as I had hoped.

Do you remember that I had used a Daily Scale to track my overall progress when I was micro-dosing? Day 30 was 2+++. Today, two months after this session, I am around a 6, which coincides with a level from my younger years. Mentally, I now have the clarity I have never previously had, and I would estimate it at around an 8, and I love it.

Physically, I am not as fit as I used to be. I was never fit, but over these last few years, as I have been less active, I am rating myself a 4. My motivation to get fit is higher than before, and theoretically, I should be sabotaging my progress now, but I'm not. I still hear a domineering inner voice asking me why I am doing this, but I think I have it under control. Thus, I would give myself an encouraging 7, since I have not tracked my progress enough to provide an accurate assessment.

My eating would be put at around a 6. I have more control over what I am eating, and when I break my rules, I don't carry that guilt around, which I have been doing for most of my life. My drive to eat is more under control than before, and my discipline, I think, has improved, but it's still not where it should be. I give myself an overall assessment of a generous 6 with great potential for improvement.

Eight Months After the First Micro-Dose...

Eight months have now passed since I first started micro-dosing, and it has been three months since I took my third Sweet Spot therapeutic dose. Here I would like to summarise how I have progressed.

Micro-Dosing Routine and Benefits

I am still micro-dosing and am sticking with the 3-day cycle. But there have been a couple of gaps because I have forgotten to take it. The longest gap I had between micro-doses was a little more than two weeks, and I suffered no forms of withdrawal at all.

In general, I find that micro-dosing is helping me to build on what I have gone through and to give me both extra energy and motivation. I see the world more positively instead of just focusing on my issues. I still have some way to go before I discover my complete self. I find that I can deal with any new problems that crop up quicker than before. And older unresolved issues no longer seem so threatening to me, and I have a more balanced mentality.

Summary of Changes

Diet: Let's start with the least effective first. My weight has dropped by only a few kilos. I still have a weakness for chocolate biscuits and snack on anything I can get my hands on. Some days, I have this in my grip, and some days, I'm in theirs. It's just the binges that are now getting in the way. Hmm, this hasn't turned out as well as I had hoped.

Physical Sensations: I feel good physically and have more energy than usual. For a small period, I had a painful lower back that stopped me from bending down, twisting and reaching for things. When I needed to do something a bit strenuous, I had to take a micro-dose of psilocybin, and this eased the pain wonderfully. Now my back is back to normal. My only problem is that my sport has come to a standstill again.

Mood: I wake up more cheerful each day and look forward to what is ahead. I am free in a way I never was before, and am more relaxed with myself and those around me. I notice some things that used to irritate me now glide off me like water from a duck's back. Instead of my brain getting 'frazzled' in such circumstances, I can hold my emotions in check.

Conflicts: Previously, specific conflicts proved too much for me, and I would 'bury' them under other non-related issues. That would start the cycle of blaming someone else. I would explode if provoked or get stressed if I felt I was about to make a fool of myself, etc. Now, I can calmly face these issues and assess them for what they are without blaming others. If something urgent needs to be addressed, I can handle it better.

If I get irritated by my stupidity or someone else's, I mostly let out a big sigh and then carry on as if nothing had happened. It helps me both in my work and my social sphere. Nobody is perfect, least of all me, and I can mostly recognise that now.

Sleep: Pretty much every night is a good night's sleep, and I am usually refreshed in the morning. Occasionally, I have a terrible night, but that's down to too much drink and food from the previous evening. At least I can now determine what gives me a miserable night's sleep and how to deal with it.

Work: My work standards have improved immensely. For the first time in my life, I am enjoying the editing phase of my work and reviewing my references to ensure my material is correct. I also think my work with my clients has improved.

Clarity of head: Before this session, I always considered what I might have done wrong, whether I had upset someone, mentally ripped someone/myself apart, found faults in myself and others, looked for arguments, etc. I now think this experiment has helped me improve my relationships with my wife, my friends, those I respect and whose company I enjoy. It has also helped me improve the quality of this book and my coaching business.

I have no destructive thoughts flying through my head anymore. I'm rarely snarling at someone or something. I am not finding faults in things the whole time, and I am not collapsing and having mini breakdowns as much (or tantrums, depending on what you want to call them). So, what am I doing differently? Well, I am essentially calmer in my mind for one thing. When I do think about things, they are more often pleasant thoughts.

This is the new me, and I love it. I can now look back on some of the good and positive things that have happened to me in the past, and I can confidently say that a significant blockage has been removed.

Dark Thoughts: Once upon a time, those dastardly Dark Thoughts were a nightly occurrence. After my NLP Breakthrough session, I managed to stop some of them, but after going to the hospital for emergency surgery and almost dying from blood poisoning, they came flooding back. Fortunately, after this third therapeutic Sweet Spot session, I have managed to stop them altogether.

I now have more interesting dreams that allow me to wake up refreshed. Amongst other things, I dream of my wife and occasionally dream about good parts in my past and my aspirations. This is one of the best things to come from taking psilocybin.

Creativity: I think my creativity has opened up entirely new horizons. My more transparent thought processes have helped me reach the standard of working today, despite room for improvement. My biggest problem is sifting through myriad ideas swimming in my head. Before, I was afraid of making a fool of myself.

Now, I don't care and can laugh about it when I do. I have started drawing as a hobby, and I love it. It's not much, I know, but I haven't put pencil to paper since art lessons in school. My main subjects then were graveyards, gravestones and anything dark and depressing. Now, I am attempting portraits, landscapes, still-life and anything that looks appealing. This, in turn, has encouraged me to design this book cover.

Humour: My dry British sense of humour has returned slightly, but with a slight difference. Previously, there used to be an edge to my voice that occasionally hurt or offended those I was teasing. Now, I have a softness in my voice when talking or teasing. I welcome this change in myself, and I'm sure others do too. I laugh more and am a little more spontaneous in my decisions. I like that I have developed a heartier and more open belly laugh that sounds more genuine than before.

Daily Scale: Hmm, after eight months, where do I stand on my daily scale? At the beginning of this experiment, I had given myself a zero, and this corresponded to the state I was living in. At the end of the 30 days, it was a little more than 2. Regarding my last assessment after Sweet Spot 2, I gave myself a 6. Taking these assessments into consideration, and given that my PTSD, addiction, depression, lethargy, anxiety, etc, are not as intense, and I have achieved new levels of creativity, clarity of thought, reconciliation with my past and new self-control and confidence.

It's not perfect, but better than I can recall, so I am now an 8. I have renewed energy, optimism, and direction. Regardless of one's past, reaching the age of fifty can be a stressful time for many regarding goals and priorities, and the choices one makes that reflect the changes in one's physical stamina. I am still finding my feet and have been lucky to have this chance of a new start to life.

What Hasn't Changed?

Although I socialise more, I'm still a bit reclusive. I don't always want people around me, as I am not a great talker. I still don't take enough time to explain things when talking to others, and often rush through what I want to say.

Unfortunately, my fitness programme has come to a halt again. Bugger!

Other New and Wonderful Experiences
I have had some new experiences since completing this third Sweet Spot.

Hiking: This has been a mini life-changing experience in its own right. Being a northerner, I have always loved the countryside in the north of England: the Yorkshire Moors, Yorkshire Dales, the Pennines, Snowdonia (Wales), and especially the Lake District. I have always loved that sensation of tranquillity; it gives me a sense of being in the middle of nowhere with the beautiful and tranquil views surrounding me. I set myself some tough challenges when hiking, and I give myself a hard time on the trail as I often have to battle against the pain that develops in my right foot, and tiredness quickly sets in my leg.

Reasons for this include stones, uneven ground, soft earth, and hard ground. It's a sensation that starts at the base of my heel as quickly as the first 100 meters or so. A small walk of about 8 to 10 km leaves me hobbling back to my destination, with each step like walking on glass.

Another problem is that I have a weak ankle and muscles in my bad leg, so I have nearly no control over foot flexibility, and even less so when bearing any amount of weight on it. My foot tends to point slightly outwards and my ankle inwards, so if I am walking on a left downward-facing slope, I am almost walking on a collapsed foot and inner ankle joint.

I can't predict how the ground will be before a walk, but I try to plan all my routes anti-clockwise around the highest point to reduce the risk of ankle pain. My next problem is that I can't walk on my toes because I don't have enough muscle strength in my leg. This means I am very heavy and flat-footed when walking on my right foot.

To aid me in walking more balanced, I have to walk with a heavy and flat-footed gait with my left foot, too. Going uphill is okay, but coming down is a nightmare. I can rely on only one leg: my left. Using this leg, I have to control my balance, weight distribution, and direction of movement, and this can quickly become tiresome and increasingly challenging as I age.

Then I have to consider where I can put my right foot without overburdening it so I can swing my left leg forward and place it on the ground without risking a fall. Going down large stony/boulder-type stones takes me a long time, even with a stick. I have to say I admire my wife's patience as she waits for me near the bottom of any decline when we go hiking together.

This summer we went hiking in The Lakes, and as with the start of every new walking season, I had to re-break in my walking boots. They are made of leather and provide reasonable support for my weak ankle, but are insufficient to allow for extreme twists or when walking on uneven, soft ground. Because my ankle bones don't sit in the correct position, the displacement causes me immense pain when they rub against the sides of the boot.

This means I need to 're-break' them by making the leather softer in time for our holiday (actually, it gives my ankle time to get used to the rubbing against the side of the boot). This year, I started re-breaking the boots several weeks in advance before we left for the UK. Bremen is very flat, so covering more considerable distances isn't a problem, but practising hill walking is, as the highest point above sea level is 32.5m.

In Bremen, it's like trying to go hill-climbing in the Netherlands—it's that flat. Anyway, I covered a lot of distance, broke my boots, and was looking forward to the Lakes. Incidentally, I need to break in only the right boot. My left foot sits in its boot wonderfully each time.

On the first afternoon we arrived in The Lakes, we decided to climb a small hill as a mini-warm up (Great Mel fell, for those who know the area) and chose to ascend the steep side. It's not that high compared to other climbs we have done in the past, and we thought we would be okay on this one for a warm-up.

First, we made our way down from Troutbeck Inn, just off the A66 where we were staying, down the narrow road to the old military rifle range, through the long grass on the old firing range and over some uneven ground before we enthusiastically hit the hill. It turned out to be steeper than we thought. My wife managed half of it, I managed a third of it, and we were both exhausted. We turned back disappointed, and I was somewhat worried about how I would cope in the following days. We quickly decided to choose a route for the next day that wasn't too long (10km) and not too high (450m at its highest point over a few kilometres).

At the beginning of the walk, I started in my old mode: hunched up with my head down, ploughing on as my wife led the way. After a couple of miles, I still felt good and relaxed and realised that some of those old negative thoughts I had always carried around were starting to melt away.

I began to enjoy my walk, and my foot didn't play up as quickly as usual. Occasionally, I stopped walking and allowed myself to take a short break while enjoying the stunning views of and around spectacular Blencathra, where we were walking. I was starting to enjoy the breathtaking scenery, unlike anything I had experienced before. I continued walking with a renewed vigour in my stride.

My foot started to hurt after a while, but I could carry on at a good pace and took the odd break when needed. It was one of the best walks I have ever done. I felt on top of the world (and not just on top of a fell). Once we returned to the car, I needed to massage my aching feet after prising my boots off, and this was the best sensation ever. I even returned to our holiday apartment in a relaxed mood and with a slight bounce in my step.

This remarkable experience continued for the next two weeks of hiking together. I had a few bad days where I had to hobble back to the car, but my mental approach differed. I wasn't in a rush to finish the route compared to many times before, yet our pace was quicker overall. I occasionally got caught up in my thoughts and had the old 'I can't do this' moment, but I found I could stop them reasonably quickly and think more constructively.

This time, over the whole holiday, nothing annoyed me other than when I cooked a lovely Madras curry in our holiday apartment and spilt it over the worktop. Although this was quickly forgotten, I realised I was not bickering over trivial things as much. My new relaxed way brought something extra into that relationship on our holiday. My wife seemed more comfortable when I was with her, and she enjoyed our holiday time together more than before.

Oh, and when I did take a micro-dose of psilocybin before walking, I had more energy, felt less pain in my heel, was clearer in my head, and thus was able to enjoy the journey, scenery, and peacefulness even more. I did several walks without micro-dosing on psilocybin, and I was a little more sluggish in comparison (a few of those days were when I had foot problems).

I've not tried stepping over the threshold while walking. I'm too unstable on my feet at the best of times, and I think this would push my luck too far. Additionally, I generally don't have enough energy to do anything physical once I step over that threshold, regardless of the dosage size.

When I consider past holidays in The Lakes, for example, I used to find excuses for not doing specific walks: Sharp Edge, Striding Edge, etc, and I dished out various reasons to help keep my ego intact. This time, though, I admitted to myself that I am not safe enough on my feet and would be a liability to others and myself, given the risk of falling if I attempted such walks. Until then, I had never been able to admit that these strenuous walks were beyond my abilities before. And here I shed a tear, as I still would love to do them.

Depression and Anxiety: I read the book *Lost Connections: Uncovering the Real Causes of Depression* by Johann Hari and found his description of the nine causes of depression and anxiety to be a great help to me. I read this book after going through my three therapeutic sessions, and it has helped me understand some of the sticking points I currently have in knowing how to behave differently.

For example, Johann explains the difference between what could be termed 'abnormal' feelings or reactions and what is 'normal' and ponders on many interesting examples. My problem was that I didn't know, or had forgotten, what 'normal' was after all these years. Once I had reviewed the differences, I realised that many of my thoughts were normal, which helped me to understand that I still have a few things in my behaviour that could be described as 'abnormal'. This new knowledge taught me how to act more appropriately and manage my thoughts more effectively.

This change didn't happen overnight, and there are still situations I must learn to recognise to respond appropriately. However, I am now much more confident in my ability to do this.

I particularly like and agree with him on how he reasons that depression is not primarily caused by chemical imbalances in the brain, but by external social events. For me, this fits in with the principles of NLP. He arrives at this conclusion after analysing the experiences of social 'disconnection' and alienation. I agree. For me, this exclusion comes from my childhood experiences.

Johann argues that people 'banding together' in social communities or, when appropriate, by using talking therapies, can often be a far more effective way of dealing with depression than taking antidepressants. This book won't help everyone to release those restrictive bonds, but it certainly provides a foundation in offering ideas for coping with that restrictive past.

An Argument that Wasn't: This was an innocuous experience that carried significant meaning for me. My wife and I were enjoying a glass of wine one sunny day during the fantastic hot summer we've just had when she made an interesting comment. But something riled me about what she had just said. My brain went through its first stages of frazzlement and was ready to kick off verbally. But the next bit of the process that would usually have led me into a one-way heated discussion was missing.

Instead, I calmly replied, 'Yeah, you're right,' and continued the conversation in a relaxed and enjoyable manner. This response started me thinking about the arguments I have kicked off and whether I had some trigger to a word, sentence, tone, or something else that set me off.

What a fantastic ten months this has been for me; my growth is only beginning. I have now reached a much higher level of mental awareness than before, and it's so refreshing. I appreciate that I still have a couple of niggling points I haven't been able to crack; however, there is a whole new world out there waiting for me, and I want to be a part of it.

Lucy

I mentioned earlier how Lucy uses psilocybin against migraines, muscle pain, and shoulder and neck spasms. Later, she felt inspired to carry out some experiments with cannabis Sativa and cannabis Indica, too. Here is what she found out:

Psilocybin

Oncoming migraine: It is always best to catch it immediately. She knows that if specific points in her neck and shoulders hurt, she must act quickly. If she must work with people, she takes a micro-dose, which helps to reduce the pain. Occasionally, it will go. If the pain remains, then she will take extra micro-doses throughout the day to keep it under some control. When she is home and has time to relax, she takes a higher dose to fight the pain. Then she needs to close my eyes before she can function again.

Migraine: Lucy starts by taking a higher dose to combat as much migraine pain as possible. Because it is so painful, she does not suffer any hallucinations, and she can function reasonably well doing basic jobs. Usually, the migraine will go away.

On some occasions, the migraine and muscle pains remain, and an hour or so later, she needs to repeat that over-the-threshold dose to eliminate it, or at least to soften the pain a little more. What I like about psilocybin is that she does not have to suffer the side effects she gets from prescription tablets, which she used to take against a migraine. She doesn't have pain in my liver and kidneys for days afterwards, and she doesn't have to suffer that groggy, tired feeling for the next couple of days also.

Muscle spasms: Light doses help to numb the pain caused by muscle spasms. If the pain eases enough, the muscles can relax for the rest of the day, and she can continue working with people. Sometimes, the pain comes back, and she will take another light dose to soften the pain again.

Sleep: If she takes a little light dose, it makes me sleepy and gives me a good night's sleep. She knows this has the opposite effect for many and makes them more awake.

Cannabis

Since beginning her journey with psilocybin, Lucy also had the opportunity to explore the effects of cannabis. In the evenings, she would take a small dose of cannabis Indica to help her sleep more soundly through the night. While it was effective in that regard, she did not enjoy the cotton wool it left in her mouth, which often made her feel thirsty.

In the early stages, while she was still gauging the correct dosage, she occasionally took too much. The result was an intense and overwhelming experience. She felt glued to the sofa, gripped by a wave of paranoia that lasted for a short while. Fortunately, this reaction disappeared after several uses and never returned.

Later, she noticed a gentle lightness in her head after consumption, which became her cue to go to bed. Reflecting on the differences between cannabis and psilocybin, Lucy found psilocybin to be gentler on her mind. In contrast, cannabis seemed to work more deeply on physical tension by relaxing her muscles.

When away from home, she preferred to carry a small amount of psilocybin in case of a migraine onset. It was more discreet and acted faster than cannabis, making it the more practical option when she was out.

How Lucy Started with cannabis

A few months after starting psilocybin, a friend introduced Lucy to cannabis. Since she did not smoke, he suggested she try making edibles. He gave her two varieties. Cannabis Indica was meant to support sleep, and cannabis Sativa provided an uplifting daytime boost. She began baking what she called cannabiscuits using a mixture of decarboxylated and non-decarboxylated cannabis butter to balance the psychoactive effects with the medicinal properties.

It took Lucy a few tries to find the ideal dose. She wanted deep muscle relaxation without a high intensity. Once she discovered that balance, cannabis became a welcome addition to her routine. Her evening biscuit eased her aching muscles and supported restful sleep, while the small morning biscuit gave her energy and focus. She described it as a coffee-like buzz that lasted into the afternoon without the jitteriness, hyperactivity or emotional swings she sometimes experienced from coffee.

Over time, she noticed reduced muscle aches and increased calmness, openness, and mental clarity. Her physical endurance improved, and she could exercise more regularly without triggering migraines or muscle tension. The benefits of the nighttime dose seemed to carry into the following day when supported by her morning Upper cannabiscuit.

Cannabis and Psilocybin

Lucy continued to microdose with psilocybin and found the combination of psilocybin and cannabis to be complementary. Each substance worked in distinct ways on the brain, the body and her thought processes. Together, they made her feel more grounded, capable and emotionally balanced. Her confidence grew, and she became better able to engage with colleagues. She even took on more responsibility at work. Her relationships with family and friends also deepened.

After several months of using both cannabis Indica and Sativa alongside psilocybin, she had almost no migraines. Only three in five months, compared to the two or three she used to experience each week. Though she still dealt with a stiff neck on some days, Lucy remained hopeful that it, too, would fade with time. She remembered years of struggling with chronic migraines that no doctor had been able to treat successfully.

Living in Hamburg, Lucy was fortunate to have access to clean and high-quality products from friends who grew their cannabis and mushrooms. She recognised that many others did not have this privilege and were often forced to rely on inconsistent and unreliable sources. Ideally, she wished she could buy these substances legally. She did not have the time or space to grow her own, and it seemed only logical that natural medicines should be accessible.

Therapy Session

After hearing from close friends about their transformative experiences with therapeutic psilocybin sessions, Lucy decided to try one herself. What surprised her most was realising how many people she had known for years had undergone these deeply healing journeys without ever speaking about them until recently.

They advised her to have someone nearby during the session who could be present in case she needed support and to reflect beforehand on a particular issue she wanted to address. Her first attempt did not go well. Something surfaced that disturbed her deeply, and instead of facing it, she turned away. She later realised that this was a mistake. Avoiding the experience had left it unresolved.

Encouraged to try again with a lighter dose a week later, Lucy was able to revisit the issue gently and bring a sense of closure. While this second session helped, it was not the kind of experience she had hoped for, and it left her hesitant to try again for some time.

Eventually, she gave it another try, this time with a different emotional focus. As the session unfolded, old memories returned, and with them came new understanding. Something heavy lifted from her. It felt like a spiritual release, a quiet but profound shift. Since that session, she has described herself as walking differently. Her posture became more relaxed, and her perspective softened. The tension in her neck eased slightly, and she carried herself with quiet freedom.

Alcohol

Although Lucy had never been a heavy drinker, she occasionally had a drink to socialise. Since beginning her experiment with cannabis and psilocybin, she found that alcohol no longer served her. It did not help her unwind. The natural substances supported a more intense relaxation and helped her understand the emotional roots of her stress rather than numbing it.

Smoking a Joint

After months of using only edibles, Lucy visited Amsterdam with her partner and decided to try smoking for the first time. At a coffee shop, she bought a pre-rolled joint. Later that day, sitting beside a canal under golden autumn light, she gave it a try. She practised holding it, inhaled slowly, and found the first few puffs surprisingly pleasant. A soft body sensation and a lightness in her head lingered for about an hour.

However, she also noticed some downsides. The smoke irritated her throat and dulled her sense of taste and smell. Food became less enjoyable until everything returned to normal the following day. She realised she still preferred edibles over smoking.

Influenza

Seven months into her experiment, Lucy came down with a severe case of influenza. She was bedridden with a high fever, body aches, tooth pain and deep pressure in her eyes and skull. Coughing aggravated her neck muscles and triggered a migraine. After two difficult days, she turned to her natural medicine cabinet. She began taking one gram of psilocybin every couple of hours and cannabis every six hours, both just over the threshold dose.

The relief came quickly. The migraine subsided, her muscles relaxed, and she could sleep. Psilocybin seemed to ease the pressure in her lungs and reduce her coughing. When coughing fits woke her, a small dose helped her settle again. She was amazed that even at higher doses she experienced no hallucinations, only calm and comfort.

Her flu symptoms had vanished twelve days later, and something even more astonishing happened. Her lifelong asthma had disappeared. She had not wheezed or coughed in days. Unsure whether to continue taking psilocybin so frequently, Lucy maintained a lower daily dose of one gram twice daily to avoid building a tolerance.

Seven weeks after the flu, she remained free of all symptoms. Her breathing was open and easy. After exercise or during stress, there was no tightness or wheezing. She felt as if she had been given new lungs. Unfortunately, her supply was running low, and she could not get more. She was forced to reduce her intake and noticed over the following weeks that her asthma gradually began to return. It was not as bad as before, but the ease of breathing she had experienced began to fade.

She wondered what might have happened if she had been able to continue. Would the asthma have disappeared altogether? Lucy remained curious and hoped to resume the experiment once she could obtain more.

Reflection
Psilocybin and cannabis had helped Lucy reclaim parts of herself she thought were lost. They brought her lightness, insight and a deeper connection to her body and emotions. She felt like a new version of herself. Her dreams no longer seemed distant, and she began exploring ideas and possibilities she had once been too afraid to consider.

To her, it was obvious. Psilocybin and cannabis hold powerful healing potential. They supported health, self-awareness and even improved relationships. Yet they remained prohibited. Lucy could not understand why she was forced to choose between pharmaceuticals that caused side effects and natural substances that helped her feel whole. It made no sense to her at all.

Thank you, Lucy, for your valuable feedback.

Sweet Spot No 4 – What Am I?

Whatever you are, be a good one.

Abraham Lincoln

At the very beginning of this experiment, there was still an immense amount of anger, hate, distrust, etc, within me, even after my NLP Breakthrough I went through, and I was somewhat sceptical about how helpful psychedelics could be for me. As each experiment was carried out, I noticed significant changes, for example, in my thinking, my attitude towards life, many aspects of my past and in discovering who I really am. That doesn't mean to say that it has been a smooth ride and an easy transition over these last ten months; it hasn't.

Since completing the third therapeutic session, I've been fortunate enough to recall some memories from my past, from childhood through middle age. Most of these were moments of happiness and reinforcing memories I had completely forgotten about. But I have also reflected on those moments that went wrong for me, and I didn't realise there was a problem then. The significant difference is that these negative memories are often accompanied by insight into how I could have behaved differently.

One crucial memory is my mother consistently encouraging me to make something of my life, and I thought I would eventually choose the wrong path. She had worried about me ending up in prison or suffering an early death after what I had gone through in childhood. This subject is something we talked about a few times before her death on how much of a burden that was for her at the time.

She never lost her self-belief in me. Mum always encouraged me to better myself and never give up fighting for what I want, even though in parallel, I have had to battle with the conflicting feeling of a lack of self-worth.

From an early age, I also learned how to be persuasive and how to influence people with my choice of words. In most cases, this has worked rather well for me. In the past, I have been offered jobs and contracts that were real challenges for me, and I was lucky enough to win the trust of others quickly.

I have been able to solve a fair few seemingly intractable problems and tolerate stagnant times where there were few challenges to be solved. Yet due to my underlying lack of self-belief, I would invariably inflict some self-punishment on myself by screwing up relationships, jobs and positions which I had been entrusted with, and sometimes this had unfortunate consequences for me.

Another problem was that I regularly saw enemies everywhere, even occasionally in close friends and family. Some continual distrust lurked in my mind, even though I liked, trusted and respected the people around me (contradictory, I know). This distrust led me to criticise, find fault with them, and put them down at (in)opportune moments. Some would laugh at me for being a prat; others would turn the situation around and make me the (deserved) fool. Others, though, would be (naturally) offended and try to avoid me.

Then there was another problem for me, and that was socialising. I preferred to remain in the background regardless of the activity. In the UK, staying in one pub for the whole evening is not always typical when going out in a group. Instead, it is usual to do a pub crawl, i.e. to have a drink in each of a series of pubs.

I hated these sessions because I can't hold my alcohol and tend to drink slower than the rest, and because each pub had a 'time limit', I ended up drunk before the evening got underway. My other problem was with my hearing. Being completely deaf in one ear made it difficult for me to converse in loud places (and still is).

Most of those friendships fizzled out, more from my side than theirs. I just never felt a part of the group. I just felt different. I've now realised that this feeling of being different stems from my childhood, but until recently, I had never really known why. Others naturally integrate, and yet, regarding me, I thought they weren't interested in what I had to say, even if they were.

One thing that has always confused me is that I never really knew how to handle other people's emotions, and this week, it is becoming more apparent why that is. I had witnessed and experienced extreme emotional, physical and persistent abuse in my younger years. Still, when it came to someone being upset or ill, I had very little or no empathy or sympathy to give them.

Even watching emotional scenes on TV, when everyone else was crying, cheering, shouting, etc., I would nod in appreciation and usually say something cold and hard or what I thought was funny, which was often inappropriate. Over time, my reactions have become tempered by experience and observation, but in many cases, I still cannot respond emotionally.

Another example that has puzzled me is that I never get emotional in sports. When watching football, for instance, fans go into a frenzy when a goal is scored. I nod, appreciate the tactics used, and watch all the others jumping around, kissing each other, and celebrating like a bunch of hyperventilating Zebedees. Initially, I would fake these emotions. Now, I've given up even doing that altogether. And for all these years, I thought something was wrong with me.

I have always loved challenging and dangerous situations, and I still do. The more troublesome something is, the calmer I remain, and I get a real buzz from it. On those occasions in which I was involved in severe accidents, I mentally dealt with the situation quite quickly, and it never came back to haunt me.

Maybe this is due to a lack of emotional depth in me, and/or that no other situation I have experienced has been as torturous as it was in my childhood, and thus, I have developed a different perspective on it. I don't know.

At some point in my life, I concluded that the only way I would be successful in my dealings with others in my job was to be cold and assertive in front of others and to be hard in my approach to problems. I then carried this over into my private life. The aim was so that I would, at least, have some control over my life. At work, I could never admit when something was going wrong or that I needed help.

This attitude was, however, self-defeating. I would get so bogged down with my self-critical thoughts that everything around me would begin to fall apart, and lo and behold, I ceased to be successful and didn't finish my tasks. In effect, I coerced myself into believing I wasn't worth the success, which became a self-fulfilling prophecy.

My way of reacting against these mistakes would be loud and brash, publicly blaming everyone else, regardless of whether they were mine. What a sad situation for me to be in. I would lie, reinterpret the facts, and conjure up a fictional situation that had never existed. And yet, all this felt right and normal to me then. I thought all those around me were thinking and doing the same. For example, this attitude brought me early success in my first job as an electrical salesman. I gained excellent sales results and achieved the best sales quotas in the shop, but I screwed the position up in my own misconstrued way.

This deceit grew along with some of my successes in the early days. I landed a series of well-paid jobs with high levels of responsibility. I would implement significant changes and introduce improvements that would benefit both staff and the company. But then, as my reputation grew, I would somehow let the self-destructive pattern repeat itself.

I would sabotage the good work I was doing and would often be moved to another, less critical project I didn't want to work on, where I felt nothing was interesting or worthwhile enough to keep me going. And if these thoughts were strong enough, I would leave the company.

Following the advice of an old boss, whom I am still grateful to, I continued my studies in post-grad business management. I quickly realised that there was a potential opening for me working as a consultant. It was one of the best career decisions I've ever made. I promptly left the company I worked for and set myself up as an independent.

The first contract I won did not go according to plan, even though I was able to help my client to some extent. Fortunately, I learnt a lot from my mistakes on that project and could complete some of my future projects with better results. Being a consultant allowed me to be me. I had to be brutal to deliver my rescue projects on time, and I was reasonably successful. This situation was ideal for me.

I never won any friends, but I got the job done coldly and calculatingly. But after staying in the same company or department for more than one contract, those destructive patterns would start to repeat themselves, I would enter into my self-destruct mode, and it would be the start of my downfall again. I quickly learnt it was better to leave on a high and start another contract elsewhere.

My other problem was that as soon as I felt something wasn't working or I had inadvertently made the sort of mistake that ordinary people make every day and either learn from or forget about due to its triviality, it triggered some self-destructive internal process that gradually wore me down mentally and turned me into my own worst enemy.

However, since going through the first three therapeutic sessions, I can now see much more clearly the causes of this.

What my father had done to me verbally and physically, I passed on orally to others. And boy, I know I can hurt with my words. Sadly, many can confirm that. It has caused me no end of problems in life, and although at that moment I wouldn't consciously know why I was doing this, there was some part of me that did, and it seemed necessary to let this verbal aggression out against them time and time again.

It is a relief to understand now what was happening in my head and why situations progressed the way they did, but I wish I had realised this many years earlier. I could have led a completely different life if I had.

Don't get me wrong, I'm not a mean and nasty person. I was merely too messed up to get my life onto the proper track, and I would try to bring others down instead of or with me. But thankfully, there have been a few moments in my life where I have managed to get some things right, to help people, and to build a few valuable relationships, which have helped me grow. In those moments, I have helped those people too. For these small moments, I am very grateful.

Another problem I have always had is never knowing what I want to do with my life. I have no clear direction; even at fifty, I still don't know how to do certain things. There are a lot of things I enjoy doing, but nothing seems quite right for me.

Even if I find something I want, I have found ways to sabotage and reject it. I enjoy writing and love working with my private and business clients with NLP. I get exceptional pleasure from seeing my clients able to get on with their lives again, so maybe this is the right thing for me.

I have few friends, and I don't mind this. As I have said before, contact and communication aren't my strong points; fortunately, my close friends know that too. They know I am a bit messed up and accept me for the way I am. I've never been the person who calls everyone a friend I have merely spoken to.

I see all people differently, and emotion rarely plays an integral part in my social interactions with them.

This is where I think things get interesting. Years ago, someone commented that I was probably a psychopath based on some reaction of mine. I know I've always been doing and saying things where angels usually fear to tread, as the old saying goes, but never thought to question whether I had any psychopathic or irresponsible tendencies. This thought returned to me about a month ago, but I dismissed it quickly. I'm not a psychopath, nor a sociopath, nor a narcissist, I told myself. I'm just messed up from the abuse I suffered as a child. Or am I?

For a simple clarification, sociopaths tend to be nervous and easily agitated. They can be volatile, have emotional outbursts and fits of rage, yet they can occasionally show empathy towards others. These people tend to be less educated and live on the fringes of society, where it isn't easy to maintain a long-term job.

Sociopaths can attach themselves to an individual or a particular group, but tend not to have moral regard or respect for society. Should a sociopath commit a crime, it tends to be haphazard, spontaneous, and unplanned. My history seems to fit into this category (minus the crime). Even the way I've written this book seems to follow this pattern.

A psychopath, on the other hand, is not able to form emotional attachments nor to feel empathy for anyone, even though they often tend to have disarmingly charming personalities. They learn to copy and mimic emotions even though they don't feel any of their own at the time. These people tend to be educated, and they can hold down a steady job as well as have long-term relationships.

Should these people turn to crime, they are very methodical and usually have contingency plans if things go awry. They are highly organised and remain cool, calm and meticulous, thus leaving very few traces, clues or evidence at the scene (again, you will find a lot of my history fits into this category too. Err... minus the crime again).

A narcissist is a little different. They lack empathy, are arrogant, self-important, judgmental and need praise and attention. However, a narcissist feels guilt and shame if something goes wrong, as I have so often experienced in my life.

From this point on, for ease of discussion, I will include narcissism, sociopathy and psychopathy under the umbrella of 'psychopath' for ease of discussion.

The thought that I have the potential of being a psychopath has grown stronger over the last few days. Rather than denying it, it seemed better to test it to determine the truth, so I carried out a recognised test. My psychopath test score was 29/40. Under the US scoring system, one is a psychopath with 30+, and in the EU, it is 25+. So, if I lived in the US, I would be classed as normal; however, in the EU, I am a psychopath. That explains a lot.

I have also taken a test for sociopathy, and this came out at 20/25. More than 16 is typical of strong sociopathic tendencies. I. Am. Shocked!

As for my narcissist test, this came out to be 31/40. It seems I'm almost a fully-fledged narcissist. I. Am. Speechless!

I now believe that it was my mixed childhood upbringing that gave rise to my predominant emotions of guilt and shame. Mum did a great job on her own in raising both my younger sister and me to be decent people. This upbringing from my mother may, in retrospect, have acted as a necessary brake on some of my otherwise strong psychopathic tendencies.

When I was younger, there were moments where I unknowingly let my developing psycho side have free rein, and it was my mother, who didn't have an insufficient bone in her body, who would point out to me that something I did or said was wrong.

Mum then explained why and how we should react as good citizens.

I suppose some psychopaths would have reacted with indifferent annoyance. Yet, I am genuinely grateful that she gave me another perspective on life, even though my parents' differing upbringings created some major conflicts within me. Mum saved me and my life from going down the pan altogether.

Typically, I would overreact to specific situations, lash out and verbally attack people if I felt it was justified, without ever considering the other person's perspective or emotions. Then I would hear my mother's voice reprimanding me, and I would realise I was wrong. However, I still couldn't recognise the emotional pain I was causing to others, and this probably manifested itself as my inner guilt or shame, I'm not sure.

This would then start a chain reaction within me: first, the justifiable reprimand and guidance from my mother, followed by my father's negative mind games about how worthless and incompetent I am.

These two inner voices would play out their conflicting dialogues. These continuous multi-records played within me for days and weeks (and sometimes over months), ending up with my father's voice gaining the upper hand in the form of self-fulfilling prophecy.

Faced with the slightest criticism from others, I would first throw out sarcastic comments, and then draw up my plans against those I saw as my enemies. Once this demon was let out, I would carefully listen to every word said and calculate its effects on the other person and would happily change direction with my plan if it helped to inflict via verbal barrages and more pain on my victim to get what I wanted. What a shit I am, eh.

Thankfully, my mother's influence has had other positive effects on me. I have avoided crime and have never initiated violence, although I have provoked a lot of people in my life and have pushed myself into some precarious corners. I do have a low snapping point, but my escalating anger seems to burn itself out before reaching dangerous levels. I have never hit a woman, and the idea of any form of physical torture against anyone or anything leaves me cold. Perhaps this is because I had experienced enough from my father, who wanted to inflict it on others who couldn't defend themselves.

Now that I better understand this cold and practically zero empathy side of me, I can better keep this trait in check. I have learnt how to talk to others without (too often) upsetting them. I have learnt how to remain calm in situations that would have previously fired me up. But what about those Dark Moments which crop up so inadvertently and unexpectedly, which, I guess, most, if not all, psychopaths, sociopaths and narcissists have to face at some point in their life?

One small step I took towards better understanding how psychopaths work was reading the excellent book *Snakes in Suits* by Paul Babiak and Robert Hare. It was as though I were reading my biography. It explained to me why I had experienced the destructive thought processes I had and why they caused me to react in such antisocial and abrasive ways.

I do believe there are some benefits to being a psychopath: I remain in control and clear-headed when dealing with my clients, when faced with challenging situations. I usually warn them at the beginning of a session that I will show no emotion, stop them from talking if I think we are losing sight of the situation, and interrupt them if they become confused or drift into talking about unrelated subjects.

This helps me get the results they need without worrying about offending them. I also find that I can readily dissociate myself from such situations, which is very helpful for me. Another benefit, although some may disagree, is that it's next to impossible to hurt a psychopath emotionally. Well, at least until

I start up my self-destructive psycho ways or someone hits a trigger point in me, then yes, I'm my own worst enemy.

I am fortunate that my wife is similar to me regarding emotion, even though she is neither a psychopath, sociopath, nor a narcissist. I love the attention she gives me, etc, but we don't need to hang around each other all the time. I like to be near my wife, but dislike physical contact with others. I feel uncomfortable with the European greeting and goodbye hugs, and still love the good old British handshake with both men and women.

I did, by the way, tell my wife that I have psychopathic, sociopathic and narcissistic tendencies once I understood the results from these tests, and asked her if she could live with that. She responded that she wasn't that surprised and still loves me just as much.

However, we both now have something to work with in dealing with those, now less numerous situations, when I get into a bit of a manipulative phase. She says I am now more attuned to her (and others) and understand certain situations more. The good news is that, thankfully, she won't leave me just because I'm all three.

Regarding my psychopathic, sociopathic and narcissistic tendencies, what parts do I want to keep? I don't want to hurt or manipulate people inadvertently, and I don't want to push people further away from me than they need to be. I want to be more relaxed and occasionally enjoy simple small talk and discussing interesting subjects without the mental clutter that typically hinders me.

A positive for me is that I can remain calm in stressful situations and respond accordingly. The question arises, though, whether it is possible to have the best of both worlds, to dissociate from a situation if need be, yet to have enough empathy to help those I am with? Theoretically and according to some psychologists, the answer is no, it's not possible. Apparently, once a psycho, always a psycho.

I now recognise, of course, that one aim of writing this book and by laying bare the conflicts and issues of my life for everybody to read is to help me work through these challenges and the new realisations about myself that these experiments reveal. My experiments with psychedelics have shown that these issues lie much deeper than I had ever imagined.

Who, in their right mind, would openly acknowledge their own psychopathic, sociopathic and narcissistic tendencies in this way after fighting against such revealing situations all their life? Huh, me, of course. At this moment in writing, I still think I am doing more damage and putting myself in a weaker situation by being this open.

I think I am also putting at risk that delicate and fragile defensive bulwark I have built up. Much of what I have fought for and against is at risk of crumbling into a pile of dust. I need to understand myself even better.

The Next Step

Today, I am ready to carry out a fourth therapeutic session focusing on my psychopathic, sociopathic and narcissistic tendencies. I want to find out what really happened to me in the past and then work through this with the hopeful result of becoming more 'normal'. I hope I can then enjoy the company of people around me and get on with the rest of my life without this constant pressure pushing me in all directions all the time.

If at worst, I remain a psychopath, sociopath and narcissist, then I would like it to be without all the accompanying guilt and shame. Releasing that alone would be excellent for me. If I better understand what kind of person I am, I may adapt my behaviour and thinking to accommodate this appropriately.

The Question

Selecting the right question is proving to be more of a challenge than I had expected. Finding the right one to ask if I hope to release those remaining old blockages and free myself further is essential. But for me, an interesting question is, will I stay a psychopath, sociopath and narcissist thereafter? If I succeed in freeing myself from the mental guilt and shame which accompanied my previous psychopathic moments, will this make me even colder, harder and more calculating? That I don't want.

I can accept that my empathy levels are deficient, but that doesn't mean I have to be as cold and hard as a typical psychopath, do I? On the other hand, I don't want to lose all of those positive and practically helpful psychopathic-associated abilities which have helped me both as an NLP coach and in many difficult real-life situations. What a dilemma I have.

When I started to think about what outcome I wanted to aim for, I discovered Andy McNab and Kevin Dutton's book *The Good Psychopath Guide*. Reading this is like finding a DIY plan for being the type of psychopath one wishes to be. Andy and Kevin discuss two kinds of psychopaths.

The bad and the good types of psychopaths are interesting to consider, too (I'm so pleased to discover this). Most people's understanding of the term 'psychopath' is limited to the (incorrect) portrayal of Norman Bates in Hitchcock's 1960s horror-thriller 'Psycho' or serial killers such as Jack the Ripper or the Moors Murderers Ian Brady and Myra Hindley.

But there are also 'good psychopaths' out there in the world. A psychopathic surgeon will perform very delicate and critical operations and, in those crucial moments, remain calm enough to save lives. In wartime, soldiers often have to make split-second decisions and having some psychopathic tendencies gives them the ability to make the correct decision under pressure that can make the difference between life and death for their comrades.

In this book, Andy and Kevin discuss aspects that make up both good and bad psychopaths and link all critical traits to a collection of dials. Turning the dial up makes that aspect more intense, and turning it down makes it less severe. They identify 12 dials: ruthlessness, fearlessness, impulsivity, self-confidence, focus, coolness under pressure, mental toughness, charm, charisma, empathy and conscience. For an average person, we could say that the dials are in the middle of the extremes, but for me to be more empathetic, for example, this dial would need turning up.

Later in their book, they explain what is required mentally in being able to change each of the dials and what mental processes are necessary for getting the best out of certain situations, as well as many other valuable tips for dealing with different stressful situations without the need to take any psychedelics.

Their book benefits those who feel they are consistently used as doormats or are too shy to respond in certain situations. It also provides plenty of tips and tricks for learning how to act appropriately and better achieve one's objectives without hurting anyone.

I now have a solid basis for preparing my question, and this has led me to consider which other psychopathic aspects I should include and how I should set each dial in a given situation.

I've had my dials tuned in to a particular value for many years and have only inadvertently changed their settings in exceptional circumstances, such as when I feel under extreme pressure when meeting new people and manipulating situations or people to get what I want. After that, the settings drift back to where they were before: cold and distant.

My Sweet Spot question needs to be formulated so that my last blockages can be removed while allowing the good psycho traits, which I don't want to lose, to flourish. I also believe one key aspect is holding me back: the irritating and restricting internal voices in my head from people in my past saying things that have tended to increase my self-doubt, even though these people I have often trusted and have helped me in many ways.

These include my Mum, sister, grandparents, aunts, uncles, cousins and close friends. If I didn't have those conflicting voices messing things up in my head, I would be free of my inhibitions.

A possible question: What do I need to work through and release to give free rein to my good psychopathic traits, which fit in with my ideas of love, life, security and health? I think there will be several interesting hours ahead for me.

The Fourth Therapeutic Trip
I prepare for my therapeutic trip using 3.6g of dried psilocybin mushrooms. After my morning coffee, I mix these revoltingly, disgustingly, horribly tasting dried mushrooms into my scrambled egg, which I can 'devour' by only allowing it to come into contact with as few taste buds as possible. I wish I had only used two eggs instead of three. Boy, that was a hard feast to get through this morning.

Warning!
Before I go any further, I would like to point out that at the end of the other three therapeutic sessions, I had started writing my notes around six to eight hours after taking my Sweet Spot dose. On this occasion, I started writing this 24 hours later. Simply put, this therapeutic trip wasn't an experience I had previously had. It was a violent vivisection of my childhood.

A lot happened in this session, and as with the other Sweep Spot sessions, I can't remember all the details, nor necessarily in the correct order. That's not a problem; the outcome is of interest. I will also leave out some specific details of what I remembered, saw, and experienced because it was intense, explicit, and very personal. Yes, it was that graphic.

Let's Begin...

Ok, now I'm feeling the psilocybin kicking in. Here goes...

So, I lay down in bed when I noticed a light sensation in my head as the psilocybin was being converted to psilocin and got to work. With my eyes closed, I wait for the first sensations to reach me. At first, I see a red brick road with red brick walls and a red ceiling. I shoot through this tunnel at a fantastic speed for about 30 seconds, and then, boof, I hit a mass of random moving colours, shapes and people I don't know, which I am fighting my way through.

It's a bit like comparing it to pushing through the Christmas shopping crowds in a busy high street. The difference is that this experience is more chaotic as they come from all directions, including from above and below. I manage to break through this barrier, and then suddenly I notice I am in my head, and it feels like an empty void except for a rusty brown wall that is too high to climb over and stretches out into infinity. A few clouds floating around me in front of the wall represent some issues I still have that I haven't been able to deal with.

A voice speaks up within me. This is the voice from my psychopathic side, and it starts telling me what is happening. "Welcome to your inner world, Neil, and I am here to help you. This experience will be good for your book, so pay attention. Look! Here is a problem of yours I have found." The psycho-voice takes me to a small patch of fog. "This is easy to solve," the voice says, and sure enough, with a click, the problem fog disappears and the problem is gone.

"Wonderful. You do know, don't you, that this is so easy for me? You don't need this therapeutic session, do you? You see, I can solve all your problems for you. Why not just get up, enjoy the day and leave me to sort this mess out for you?" I even get out of bed, inclined to believe what this psycho-voice is telling me.

But when I start thinking about it, I realise I have several hours ahead of me and decide to distrust this domineering advice by lying down again. "And look, Neil," the voice continues, "here's another problem we can eliminate. You can put this success of mine into your book, too." And sure enough, boof, the problem-cloud disappears.

This goes on for about half an hour. The voice guides me around my brain, cracking several remaining problems. I start to get miffed as this session is supposed to be dealing with the psychopath within me, instead of it controlling the session. I know I must overpower the voice somehow, but I am unsure how. My only thought is that the only way to overwhelm it is for the psilocybin's effect to increase in intensity. I can only wait until, and if, that happens.

After some frustration with my inner psycho-voice, I get up and head for the sofa in the living room because I am suddenly hit with an intense wave of nausea. It's the worst one I have had to date. I place the cushions at the end of the sofa, pull a blanket over myself and get comfy.

Please note that during all my other therapeutic Sweet Spot sessions, I have always had the option of deciding on whether to continue to approach the problem in front of me or to pass it by. Yet, in this and the other scenarios I'm about to describe, I saw no problem until I was thrust into it, and I had no choice but to go along with it. Here's what happens…

Before I let out my first proper breath, sprawled out on the couch, I am suddenly assaulted by a barrage of punches, kicks, flying feet and slaps that are nevertheless being buffered by something: buff, buff, buff. I am being pummelled by something huge and angry, and accompanying this is the feeling of being drawn into some bound physical fight on the sofa. The main target of the attack, whatever it is, is smothering me, and occasionally, a swinging fist or a flying foot makes painful contact with me.

This torrent has no escape, and I also struggle for air. My arms and legs are pinned against me against something soft as I writhe against this torrent of abuse. My head is trapped, as though it is being held during that barrage. I'm not sure whether I start to lose consciousness or enter a deeper aspect of the trance, or go numb as a result of breathing problems.

Either way, the barrage of physical abuse eases up after what seems like a long time, and I sense the attacker gets up and walks away. I need several minutes to calm down and regain my breath.

Upon reflection, it's easier now to describe what happened. My father was attacking my mother, and she was protecting me from his incessant beatings. I couldn't breathe too well because my head was being pulled tightly into her body as she tried to defend me. Mum didn't have time to put me somewhere safe before he launched into his cowardly tirade.

It was my Mum's body that dampened most of the strikes. The ones I felt were the lashing fists and swinging feet that connected against me, which Mum couldn't block. I am over a year old, maybe eighteen months old, and I am in this scenario. What I am not sure about is whether this was just one assault I was reliving, or it was a collage of actual attacks that we endured over some time.

After getting my breath back, I go to the loo. In Germany, it's typical for men to sit down to pee, and I've grown accustomed to it. Afterwards, I stood up. I either lose my balance or something pushes me to the floor, and the beatings start up again. I have no control over what is happening to me. Yet, I either have some temporary black-out, go deeper into the trance, or the intensity increases such that I no longer recognise my surroundings.

My arms and legs are lashing out, and my head is swinging from side to side each time one of his hard fists or feet strike me. I don't notice the cold ceramic floor tiles that are unrelenting and hard, just like the ones on the side of the bath. This time, the abuse is directed against us both, but then it eases up. I see my Mum's terrified face as her thin, bedraggled body is yanked away, and the attack is now directed at her. She is looking at me, watching me to see if I don't get hurt as she is being beaten and abused.

I try to go to her, but I can't move. I am physically lying on the bathroom floor, shaking and shivering as I cry out to her. I reach out, but I can't touch her outstretched hand. That image of my Mum's worried face is still etched in my mind as he continues to attack her. I can't get rid of that image. And neither do I want to. I want to remember what happened and use it as a source of strength for my remaining future, remembering her unconditional love for me and recognising what she went through to give me a chance at life.

Again, after thirty minutes or so, the barrage dies down. He backs off, and my mother remains motionless on the floor for a while before she closes her eyes and curls up into a ball. Then Mum disappears. After several long minutes, I get my breath back and my orientation too. I pick myself up, stagger towards the bed, and crawl under the duvet. I'm unsure whether I want to go through something like that again.

Something else worth pointing out here is that I have none of the typical psychedelic dizziness and no other hallucinations usually associated with a trip between these attacks. The psychedelics seem to be no longer affecting me, except for that intense sensation of nausea, which has remained with me from the moment I left the bedroom.

Back under the duvet, I close my eyes and I notice that the psychopathic voice within me has gone completely. Not reduced, nor changed, but gone. There is no domineering voice telling me what to do. Relieved that it has stopped, I realise that I am now twenty-two years of age. It is at this point in my life that the psychopath in me has finished its apprenticeship through me and graduates with total power over me.

I lay back and try to think what happened at that age, which caused this psycho-transition. I am suddenly pulled through something too quickly to observe what it is, and I am thrust into the Universe. Suddenly, I am surrounded by many spirits guiding me.

They gave me a whistle-stop tour and explained how the Universe works and how it will help me in the future now that I am a part of it. This is a fantastic sensation, and it makes me feel good knowing I am no longer alone.

I see various dead and alive spirits who are essential to me: my wife, the gatekeeper, Mum, both my grandparents and friends, and some others I don't seem to recognise just yet. In the blink of an eye, they first merge into my dissociated spirit and then are absorbed into me. What an inspiring sensation this is that washes through me. I lay there and enjoy my newfound freedom and oneness, and I want this super sensation to carry on in eternity.

I notice I need the loo again. I get up and tootle to the bathroom in a better and more relaxed mood, having just gone through what I have in the Universe. I sit on the loo, take aim, fire and miss. How can one not hit such a wide pan opening when sitting on top of it? A little miffed, I clamber down on my hands and knees to clean up the mess. Having finished doing that, and just as I'm about to stand up, I am knocked to the floor by another barrage of abuse lashing out at me.

Like the last time, I start lashing out with my arms and legs. My head and body swinging from side to side, trying to avoid that endless barrage of punches and kicks. This time, it is just him against me, and I take each and every punch and kick and every nasty word the bully throws at me. Boy, those punches and kicks really hurt, and I'm crying with fear for my life.

After about half an hour, the attack eases up, but it takes a little longer before my aching body can sense the cold, hard tiles underneath me. I must have been around four or five years old in this scenario. Again, as with the last attacks, what I am not sure of is whether this was just one assault I was experiencing, or it was a collage of assaults merged into one.

Exhausted, I return to the living room and collapse on the sofa. For about an hour, I lay there motionless and exhausted. It's usually time for some reflection, the philosophical phase, but not much is going through my mind. After that hour passes (about five hours after first taking the psilocybin), a violent force thrusts me down against the sofa again, and I am lashing out against another torrent of physical violence against me.

As usual, it consists of kicking, hitting, slapping, and shouting abuse. Like the last time, I was alone with him, but I was around six this time. This torrent goes on for about twenty minutes until the barrage eases up, stops, and then this brave man that can only attack small babies, children and defenceless women walks away.

This time, it is a physical strain on me, and I just lay there motionless on the couch for over an hour. My body hurts; my ribs and my stomach aches from the pummelling, and the nausea still hasn't eased up at all. My face feels flattened, my arms are weak, my back aches, and my legs and hands shake from the remains of the adrenaline rush I have just gone through.

Once I get my breath back, I start to feel physically weak, and the nausea in my stomach is still intense. I am breathless and disoriented. I don't feel too good, and I think I need help. I stagger off the sofa and wander around the living room, wondering what to do. After a while, I decided to call an ambulance for help.

But after some thought, I don't. Psychedelics are illegal in Germany, and the last thing I want is to have lots of questioning in the hospital from the police, so I finally end up telling myself that what I am going through is part of the session. The risk of going to the hospital isn't worth it. After a long while, I lay back down and started to breathe more deeply and slowly. Gradually, I calm down, my body relaxes, and my tension eases. I'm fine. No ambulance needed.

Slowly, the effects of the psychedelic start to wear off, and I gradually come back to my senses. Other than sensing that battered feeling through my whole body, I notice that the domineering psychopathic voice I had at the start of the session and which had accompanied me for the whole of my adult life has completely vanished and hasn't returned since it disappeared after an earlier beating.

There is now another new inner voice there. It's softer, friendlier, and more helpful. I'm unsure whether the same voice has changed or whether it is a different voice. Perhaps my original inner voice has finally managed to set itself free. I try to think of situations that might trigger a psycho response, and thankfully, there is no reaction. It leaves me in peace; all I have is silence in my mind and around me. Wonderful.

After a while, I started to feel the texture of the sofa against my hand. I've never noticed that before. It has texture. I get up and touch the wooden coffee table, the clothing, the duvet, and a towel. It's as though I recognise texture for the first time. Then I look around me and everything seems nearer, like I am a part of it, and it is a part of me. I wander around our apartment and notice how connected I feel to everything around me. I now feel I am a part of the world and no longer detached from it. This is a new and weird sensation for me. Nevertheless, I like it.

I lay back on the sofa because this session has left me exhausted. I need to get my breath and energy back. With my eyes closed, I think about various situations I have been in which have involved my psychopathic side and how this now makes me feel inside. I feel a part of me is missing. It's a bit like a chunk of something has been ripped out of me and has left a void inside me. It was as if that second psycho-personality, which had had control of me for all those years, had been trying to keep control of the situation during my trip to avoid its demise. It had decided what I should do, and I (unthinkingly?) followed it.

Now I feel associated with the world and with life around me. I now recognise how I have been completely detached from the world surrounding me for most of my life. Not only that, previously, there had been a kind of feeling of superiority which both pervaded and surrounded me, as if I were an ultimate God and was better than everyone else, even though deep down I knew I wasn't. Confusing, isn't it?

Imagine what this feeling of newfound freedom is like. I've lost a part of me that has dominated my life for the last fifty years and which had turned me into something I wasn't. Yet, it's gone. Completely. I know it's just 24 hours since completing this session, and only time will tell how I am after I re-enter the real world with all its daily hassles once again.

That evening, after the session, I went to bed early. Throughout the night, I dreamed of various things. I don't know what exactly, except that these are the most reassuring, friendly, and comforting dreams I have had since starting this experiment. Probably it is my conscious mind realising it's now on its own and doesn't have an oppressive master anymore. I sleep well, but not brilliantly.

My body and neck are still aching from all that thrashing and pummelling. I ache all over. Even on the day after the session, my neck is still hurting. However, my hurting body muscles have released a little. I'm still tired and I need to conserve my strength.

Before I went through my last violent beating, I thought about the many children and women who are brutally abused and beaten up badly and regularly, by violent people who think they have the right to take a part of their personality and soul away from other children's lives.

It became clear to me that I needed to do something to help these people escape from such abuse, but I wasn't, and still aren't, sure what that should be. However, I am sure this will become clear to me at some later date. Our governments do very little to protect their folk, and charities, personal networks, etc., are often left to do what they can.

What Do I Think Happened in This Sweet Spot Session?

Hmm, where do I start? Before I carried out this last session, if someone had asked me whether psychopaths are born, I would have probably said yes. Maybe some of us are indeed born that way. One example I can think of is the fantastic fictional book and film *We Need To Talk About Kevin* by Lionel Shriver, in which Kevin is born to a good family but has a nasty, psychopathic streak in him.

I don't know how true this is to life, but it raises that valid question. Now, I think we are all born beautiful babies, just needing love and attention and wanting to give it back by putting our complete trust and faith into those who should know how to care for us. Yet, for some poor unsuspecting child, there's a role-model (or role-models) that abuses this trust by manipulating, beating, hitting, slapping, kicking and shouting soul-destroying things at that defenceless, trusting and innocent little child for some incomprehensible reason.

Eventually, this vulnerable child reaches a threshold point where it gives up hope of obtaining that much-craved love which it needs, and some detached personality replaces this craving through the need of self-preservation. In some or maybe even the majority of cases, the child then spends the rest of its adult life ranging from quietly defending itself to wreaking its vengeance on the world and those who cross its path, searching for that impossible-to-find inner peace and acceptance.

As I have said before, if it wasn't for the love and dedication my mother had given me as a child, I think I would have gone off the rails entirely if I were left in my father's hands. Mum gave me my life and direction, and she saved my life. I realise this more than ever now I have worked through this session, and this is now helping me to bring a fuller and deeper closure to my grief following her death three years ago. I am sure it will take me a while to make my way through this, but I will do it in good time.

Just as that violence and abuse from my father, along with my mother's dedicated love, created me into a confused psychopath, being able to re-live that experience the way I have has helped me to re-programme the neurons in my brain and remove the damage it did to me as a child.

It has now allowed my true self to be set free. It may take me a while to live with this new freedom comfortably, yet I am already noticing differences in this very short time frame. I am typing this with a different mentality. I am even more relaxed, no longer feel pressure to complete this book, and have no doubts or anxieties flying through my brain like before. I am planning what I must do for my future, and quietly getting on with it. This change, for me, is one form of true freedom.

Would I do it again? Hmm, this therapeutic session was very intense. But yes, it was worth it, and I would do it again if it would help me deal with another issue as fierce as this. The only difference is that the next time, I would probably have someone nearby, should I start to develop those breathing and disorientation problems again. I've now faced and dealt with my past, and this hefty blockage has now been released, and I've removed the psychopath from within so that I can finally be myself.

Some other minor issues have remained with me through the last three sessions, but they seem to be gone too. I guess time will tell if this is the case. My inner body feels relaxed now, and my heart is quietly working under no duress. My mind is calm. Wonderful! Finding this new inner peace is worth every punch and kick I endured yesterday.

Three Days Later...

It's now three days later, and I am excited to share my new experiences. Firstly, my physical strength and stamina are almost back to their pre-Sweet Spot four levels, but I still can't do anything too strenuous as I get out of breath quickly. Each day, I manage a little more.

My mind is still and quiet; I am at peace with myself, and it's terrific. I'm even thinking about everyday things in a completely different way. One example is that when I'm thinking about certain things that involve other people, I can step into their shoes and consider their viewpoint to a degree I never thought possible.

A softer and rounder inner voice helps me consider many other perspectives without hinting at another agenda. It is like me being in complete control of myself and my thoughts, giving me a new lease of life. This is a new experience for me, and one which is adding a new dimension to my life.

I've tested out a couple of those tough nuts that I couldn't crack in the first three Sweet Spot sessions, and they have gone completely. And, no, I don't think the psycho in me cracked them. I did this myself under the significant influence of psilocybin. If you don't mind, I would like to leave these descriptions private, as they are somewhat personal to me and beyond this book's scope.

There is still a void within me; however, with each passing day, this sensation becomes less intense and is replaced by more natural emotions. In this case, time is a great healer.

I've done a couple of tests to determine whether the psychopath in me is lurking behind some grey matter somewhere, and I've allowed myself to be provoked by those I know that can wind me up, yet, there's no adverse reaction within me whatsoever.

When I did these tests, allowing myself to be wound up by those I usually avoid, my brain was at first confused, but quickly responded and reacted in a relaxed and calm manner. I even replied with some neutral comments I would have never considered. My freed brain is now better able to process and control incoming information.

Have I lost those functional psychopathic skills? I think the experiences from my past are still there in my memory banks, and I hope to use them when needed. One evening, I encountered a pushy person at a small public event I visited to listen to some live music, and I was able to handle the situation with ease. This created a win-win situation for us, not just for me, unlike my typical approach. It may be a while before I know for sure, but I sense there is a new, good person/psychopath in me.

So, how can I test this theory? Suppose I look at the questionnaires out there. In that case, they are all written to determine whether we are psychopaths only, and I can't find anything official which differentiates between being a good or a sinister psychopath other than Andy's and Kevin's book. Either way, in the next couple of days, I will repeat the test I have done before and as objectively as I can, I will answer the questions. This goes for the sociopath and narcissist tests, too.

Although it is now only three days after completing my fourth session, I feel justified in assessing myself on a Daily Scale 9. I am currently experiencing and living a life I have never had before. Words can't express what this means to me, to be completely free. So, why only a 9 and not a 10? Because I'm still going through a mental transition phase and I have only 1 point left on the scale, just in case I feel even better than I currently am. I realise and love the difference, but my state changes daily, and I don't know what will happen to me in the long run. I need to wait until these changes stabilise within me before giving a final assessment.

Seven Days Later...

Where do I start? Considering all these continual changes within me, it has been a fantastic week. The first thing I want to reflect on again is how relaxed and calm I am. My thoughts are so at rest, and I enjoy simply 'being' and living for the present. This relaxed 'here and now' sensation has never lasted with me for more than a few minutes at the most.

However, I also think about the various simple things and daily activities I need to do now or in the future. The difference is that I am no longer distracted by those internally conflicting voices. They're gone, giving me a fantastic new sense of freedom.

I have, in short, lost that psychopathic voice that was continually blabbering, scheming and complaining in my ear. It's gone! Every day, I test to see whether it has found its way back, to make sure. I have put myself in provocative situations to get a reaction, but I have nothing.

It's gone. I am now planning the following stages of my life, including new projects, etc, and my thoughts and ideas flow unhindered by all the scheming machinations and dark fantasies that I used to have.

I have had the opportunity to test myself recently when someone belittled me. Previously, I would laugh if it was aimed at someone else and scowl when it was focused on me. On this occasion, I wasn't riled at all and even threw in a few new ideas so that they could continue to tease me.

This is super!

I decided to carry out the same psychopathic test again, which I had taken before. The last time I scored 29/40, and this landed me in the category 'psychopath' according to the EU norm. This time, I had to think hard about each question and mentally test how I would react if I were in that situation now.

My score came out to be 8/40. However, I would love to have this verified by an expert. It is the first whole week of this new me, and it seems to be a promising start. Unfortunately, there are no tests out there to determine whether a psychopath is no longer a psychopath, so I may never really know the true therapeutic extent of the benefit from this fourth Sweet Spot session.

The other problem is that a couple of questions in the questionnaire are linked to the past. I need to refer to the past in answering the questions as though I am reflecting on them for the first time and assuming that I have always been the way I am now.

I have also repeated the sociopath test. Again, I have reflected on my answers, the way I am today, and I assume I have always been like this when considering the questions from my past. My previous score was 20/25. This was a cracking score for a sociopath. This time, I scored 6/25, falling short of the sociopath category. Thankfully. So, am I no longer a sociopath?

Again, I don't know if this is true. Time will tell. One social change I notice is that I am at peace with my company and don't need to be around others the whole time. And when I am with others, I enjoy their company, with no strategic thoughts flying through my brain and no intrusive mental distractions preventing me from concentrating on how and what people are saying.

Also, I would become anxious if I did something wrong, regardless of how small, such as spilling my drink or letting out some inappropriate comment I wish I hadn't. I would become extremely worried about how people might react or what they might think about me. Now I calmly wipe up my mess, add a quick apology (if needed) and carry on as before. Or if someone is offended by something I said, I can reflect on my choice of words and say something to reassure them, as needed and then carry on with the conversation.

The other thing I have noticed is that I'm more participative in conversations. This is also because I can now better listen to and concentrate on what is being said. What a release this is for me. As with the psychopath test, I will retake it in a couple of months to see whether this remains reasonably constant.

And I have repeated the narcissist test too. Before this fourth therapeutic Sweet Spot session, it was 31/40 (yep, an almost fully-fledged narcissist). This time it is 4/40. According to this result, I am no longer a narcissist.

Has this fourth Sweet Spot session had such an effect on me? Just like the other two, I need to repeat the narcissist test in a couple of months. A question arises, I am not sure how to answer; which was the predominant in me, the psycho, the narcissist or the sociopath?

Also, how does an ex-psychopath/sociopath/narcissist function once these traits are no longer there, when compared to a person who has never had any of these three traits? Unfortunately, I couldn't find any information to help me with these questions.

Another point I notice is that my speaking voice mirrors the state of my inner thoughts. If there is an interesting point I want to make, I now do so in a more relaxed and less hurried manner and a friendlier tone. I occasionally stumble over my words, but it's nothing like it used to be.

My wife says she notices a big difference in me, too. She finds me more relaxed and easier-going, and we have more fun together. Much to our pleasure, our discussions tend to be deeper and more interesting than before. She says she finds it easier to talk to or ask me about something because I can listen better and am more eager to help if she needs it.

If I can't, I am more prepared to say so, and we both accept the outcome much better. I can devise alternatives to achieve what I can't do directly at that moment, and together we can often find new ways to achieve what we want. My wife says she feels more relaxed and confident around me now and has noticed this ever-increasing transformation in me since starting my experiment.

This is the cherry on top of the cake. I wonder how she has put up with me all these years.

Regarding sports, I know it is still a bit early to come to definite conclusions, but things are different. I've started doing the *Insanity* workout again. I had let this slip a bit for a few weeks before my fourth Sweet Spot session. Now, I am more focused and able to follow the instructor on the DVD. Previously, I would often get so lost in my thoughts, etc., that I would forget which exercise I should be doing, and I was frequently left behind.

Not only that, but my constant, intrusive, psycho thoughts would physically exhaust me, such that after a while, I would give up on doing sport altogether. I am pushing myself harder now and can concentrate fully on the moment. I'm still exhausted after completing a session, and of course, I know I am not fit or young enough to keep up with the impressive fitness fanatics in the DVD sessions. As it's a nine-week fitness programme, I shall see what happens over the next few months.

I want to link this experience with my eating habits, which have changed completely. I first noticed the difference one day when I popped out for a cup of coffee to have a break from my work desk. I usually eat a slice of cake with it, but I just ordered the coffee this time. The waitress asked me if I had forgotten to order the cake. Even though it has only been seven days since finishing my session, I have effortlessly avoided eating biscuits, cake, chocolate, or anything sweet.

I have also unwittingly stabilised my main diet. It just needs minor fine-tuning, and I'm considering how best to do this. I will review my eating habits again in a few months to see how lasting the effects have been.

I am now sleeping so effectively and contentedly for six to eight hours at a stretch, and it's terrific! My dreams are so light that sometimes I wonder whether I have been dreaming. My life has no real stress as it used to, so I don't know how I will react once my circumstances change.

Either way, I wake up refreshed and jump out of bed to get on with the day ahead. When starting this experiment, I never dreamed I could achieve this, maybe because I never had so much as a glimpse of what I could have been as I do now.

Throughout this experiment, I rated how I felt on a Daily Scale. Remember, I considered that the value 7 represents my lifetime best experience. I have reserved the maximum value of 10 to indicate that I have reached my limit of positive change. Around the sixth day after completing the fourth Sweet Spot, the change in me is so great that I feel I should raise my daily-scale value from 9 to 10+.

I would love to use a higher number to reflect the new changes within me because I have far exceeded my wildest dreams and wishes, and it is fan-bloody-tastic! Only time will tell whether this change is permanent or a short-lived wonder.

One thing that hasn't changed is my emotional level. On the one hand, I'm more relaxed, playful, reflective and proactive. However, I am still rather cold emotionally. I now think it's just the way I am - emotionally cold. There's no planning, manipulation or revenge involved in my thought processes.

I think about what needs to be done in a cool, calm and logical way as I search for my way forward. Am I bothered? No, not really. I now realise I've been emotionally cold all my life, but I have now come to terms with the way I am. Perhaps one day all this will change again, and the evil psycho in me will return (I hope not). Again, I'll know for sure once a few months have passed.

In summary, since this fourth Sweet Spot, I have become a completely different person. I am now a freer man after more than fifty years of mental imprisonment. I know these experiments are illegal and could get locked up for doing them. But it's worth the risk.

What is essential in the old grey matter is that I am free as a bird, and nothing can take that experience away. Not my father, not the government and not even the threat of prison from some old-fashioned psychedephobic judge.

By finally ignoring the government's advice, I have my life and sanity back. What more could I wish for? Maybe if my government had been there for me and for the people they were supposed to represent in the first place, instead of feeding their narrow business-biased greed, I and thousands, if not millions, like me wouldn't have had to suffer the paralysing traumas which have decimated our lives.

Since carrying out this last Sweet Spot session, I'm lucky that my Daily Scale is still at a 10+, and the changes I notice within me each day should push this figure much higher. I am already getting on with my new life with the help and guidance of my wife and the Universe. The boundaries of my previous life have been obliterated, and I now have my new life in front of me.

My previous Sweet Spot therapeutic sessions have opened up the potential for a new direction and way forward in my life. Each day feels like a wondrous adventure in learning something new and discovering what I can give back to society. We never know what is around the corner, and life continues regardless of what happens to us.

A relief is that I can now laugh freely and enjoy the simple things around me. It's not that I don't have my horrific history and memories anymore, I do. They will remain with me until I die. But the difference is that I now have the inner strength and resources to override them, so I can enjoy and live my life fully and view the past as the past and nothing more.

We owe it to our Spirit or Subconscious, or whatever you want to call it, to live our physical life to the full, to give to and help those less fortunate than ourselves and to make this a safe and secure place to live in so that we and future generations can thrive and live together peacefully.

Three Weeks Later...

By the beginning of this third week, I noticed my thoughts were all over the place. It feels like a lot of old anger is building up within me, and it wants to break out and be free. Fortunately, I have a seldom-used punching bag and let all my frustration out into that. It has helped me calm down a bit.

On the whole, though, it feels as if the effects of this fourth Sweet Spot session are still working through creating changes and destroying old processes within me, and this is a step in the right direction.

Recently, I was involved in an unexpected situation in which I would typically have reacted with verbal aggression. Instead, I remained calm and left it as it was. I believe I am now better able to understand what happened. An aggressive trigger, which would typically have determined my reaction, seems missing.

At the same time, I rationalised over positive alternatives to avoid an altercation. Instead of being motivated by self-interest, I could see things from the other person's perspective.

My eating habits have greatly improved over the past three weeks, and I have lost 4kg. I am not tempted by anything sweet. Once, I yearned for something 'delicious', but after a quick search at home, I found nothing. After a few minutes, I had forgotten about it, and the craving didn't return. Earlier, I would have rushed out to the shops to get a pack of biscuits or a bar of chocolate or two and woofed them down.

This is fantastic, I could accept that I didn't want or need it and do something else instead. I know my wife has a stash of biscuits in her office, yet I have no desire to find them. My regular eating habits have also changed, in that I am eating less with my main meals, too. As soon as I notice that I've had enough, I stop. This is wonderful. Previously, I would clean my plate each and every time.

My daily activities have changed too. I am more focused and concentrated than before, and my working sessions last much longer. Much to my wife's delight, I am physically more active and completing more odd jobs around the house than before. It's all so much easier when that inner psycho-voice isn't continually shouting at me in my head. Previously, I would have muttered to myself if I had to do a job that didn't benefit me somehow. Now, I'm even searching out jobs that need doing, regardless of what they are.

My sport is still going well, and the fact that I have lost that 4kg makes it more of a pleasure to do. I'm ploughing through *the Insanity DVD course again,* and this time my sessions are different. I'm putting more effort into each activity I need to do, and I reflect on the session differently. Instead of complaining that there is only a certain amount of time left, I am fully immersed in it and count it down with more motivation. I'm exhausted afterwards, but it now seems worthwhile.

I met up with a good friend, with whom I am usually a bit reserved for various reasons. This time, I didn't give a toss. We had a few drinks, a good laugh and a fantastic sing-along to some songs. I cannot sing at all, and it even hurts my ears when I do, but I didn't care, I belted them out… 'Mama… Just killed a man. Put a gun against his head…' Ahem, where am I? Ah, yes. I pitied my friend having to listen to my singing, ha-ha! The last time I did something like that was more than 18 years ago, after too many drinks.

Three weeks after starting this last experiment, I can still detect a small part of my former psychopathic side. I'm a little colder in my thinking, which is more logical and focused. Yet I am considering things more actively and planning more, although it is significantly less calculating this time. The most considerable difference, however, is that I don't have that stern voice bawling at me in my head. That's gone.

If I had done something wrong, I used to feel guilty or ashamed about it. This feeling of intense shame has gone too. Now I can reflect clearly on what has gone wrong, why and what I need to do. Not just from my perspective but from the viewpoint of others, too. And I like this. It could be that this Sweet Spot session has cracked the narcissistic and sociopathic sides in me, but not the psychopathic side. Sociopathically speaking, I feel much more open and relaxed around others. However, I'll wait a couple of months until I complete the tests again before giving a final verdict.

One Month Later…
It just gets better with each passing day. Let me run through my changes in no particular order of preference.

My aggression has gone, and I don't need the punching bag anymore. I guess that it was previously necessary to release all that pent-up anger that had accumulated in me over all those years, but the fourth Sweet Spot session has eliminated the need for this. I'm much calmer and more patient than before, although I sometimes get a little irritated with other people, things and myself, but hey, who doesn't? The main thing is that I now have it under control.

My weight is continuing to drop. At the end of these five weeks, I have not made any significant changes, and I have lost a total of 7kg (15.4 lbs). Eating has suddenly become a pleasure, so I can easily decide when and what to eat.

One Month Later

Near the end of this first month, I had an unplanned pig-out day and ate quite a lot. I felt I had been eating too little, and suddenly my body cried out for more food. It was a one-off day event, and my eating has returned to normal. I thought this would be an issue, but fortunately, it isn't.

Good, too, is that with my weight loss, the risk of having a heart attack has reduced from high to medium based on a scale for my age and weight. This is undoubtedly an achievement. The other great, but minor, achievement is that I have dropped a waist size in my trousers. Finally!

I'm still active with my sport and have completed the first part (the first four weeks) of the fitness course *Insanity*. The second part lasts one week, and I am in the middle. Next week, I will start the really 'insane' part, which lasts four weeks. I'm still not doing yoga, mainly because I'm exhausted after doing the *Insanity* routines. Let's see what happens in the future...

Outside of the home, I am more active, meeting up more often with friends, and enjoying socialising more. It's lovely now that the psycho part that was in me doesn't take over. I'm even enjoying being with larger groups of people. I still find it hard to participate in group conversations, but that is more down to having only one functioning ear.

I like reviewing my past because I can still remember what happened. This is the same when I think about what may happen in the future, in terms of the goals that I have achieved and would like to achieve, but I now have more control over when that happens and when it should stop.

The new clarity in my thinking still surprises me each day. I love being able to think about what I want without any mental disturbances or the need to devise sophisticated strategies for everything. It's wonderful. It even positively affects my mood, which seems to improve. I have noted improvement every day since my last Sweet Spot session.

Not only that, but I also feel entirely associated with my surroundings and the people I meet. I feel as though I am a part of this life, and I know I am playing along with it, and it is playing along with me. I am connected to the world and the Universe. Wonderful!

As for Dark Thoughts, I haven't had one dark or mildly disturbing thought at night for a long time. I sleep like a baby, I wake up refreshed and, on most days, I jump out of bed first thing, ready to go. On other days, I enjoy a few minutes longer in bed without any feelings of guilt. I remember saying at the beginning of the book that if those Dark Thoughts occurred only a couple of times a week, I would be happy. Believe me when I say I'm ecstatic with the current results.

My patience levels have shot through the roof. Previously, I would lose my patience quite quickly when I got frustrated with challenging people, and yet here I am, remaining calm and helping people where I can. The situations are not critical in themselves; how I react counts. Another way of putting this is to go with the flow of what is happening around me and enjoy it.

It's like taking a back seat in life for a while and observing it while I am enjoying myself. Did I say, 'enjoying myself?' Yes, I am enjoying my life more than I have ever done before. This freedom has no boundaries, meaning I can explore to my heart's content. And that's what I am doing. I sometimes feel like a kid in a sweet shop with all these new activities I am participating in, absorbing what is going on and remembering it.

This was a wonderfully significant experience, which made me so happy. I am enthusiastic about the sequel to my life.

Now to the interesting question of whether I have turned back into a psychopath. My previous score was 8/40, and the repeat test five weeks later is 12/40. There is a slight increase, but it is still much less than before. I'm not surprised, as I have noticed that a few weakened tendencies have returned these days. This is the only negative from all I have experienced so far.

As for the narcissist test, my last score was 4/40, and this time it is 5/40. A point difference doesn't worry me at all, and I firmly believe that my old narcissistic tendencies have gone altogether. I have no shame or guilt flying through me at all. I think, I decide, and I respond. If it's a wrong decision, I don't feel bad or guilty, but I do look at what I need to do to make it right, and if possible, correct it.

Now comes the sociopath test. The last time I scored 6/25, this time it is 5/25, a point lower. I'm more social, organised, relaxed, and friendlier; this is a significant step forward.

My other point of interest is on my daily scale. After two weeks following my fourth Sweet Spot, I rated it as 10+ as I can't go higher and theoretically, my life couldn't get any better. After these five weeks, I would put this value even higher, if I could (I can, but I'm not going to). Probably a 10 followed by another 10 +'s! Even that seems conservative in comparison to how I really am. Maybe a score of 20+ would be better to highlight my current experience. Perhaps I should have increased this scale further.

Two Months Plus One Week Later...

Around the end of the first month and at the start of the second month, I started having some mental issues regarding some of the small psychopathic parts I wanted to keep. I had unintentionally started a couple of conflicts for no reason at all. How do I know it was related to a part of the psychopathic side I wished to keep?

I thought I was being manipulated somehow, but after some reflection, I wasn't. This thought of possible manipulation bothered me, as it has happened several times. Now I don't know what to do with this remaining psycho part within me, and not only that, I don't like it anymore. Can I eliminate it, or do I now need to accept that a part of it will always remain with me, causing occasional problems for the rest of my life?

A few days later, I felt ill after working in the cold weather for too long without enough warm clothing, and I was hit with a slight fever, lower back pains, and a constant headache. The first night, I couldn't sleep. The following day, Lucy gave me a couple of cannabis Indica biscuits to eat that evening to help me out. She told me that if I ate half of one, I would sleep through the night, which should be enough for four nights. Worried I wouldn't sleep, I ate them both.

That night, I slept for around seven hours solid, which helped me recover from my cold, and I felt a lot better the next morning. But more significant was the experience that left me completely and utterly impressed. The two canna-biscuits threw me into a trance, and a deep one at that. I had no tripping effects like with mushrooms and was immediately launched into the Universe, where a discussion ensued with my spiritual supervisor.

We discussed those few remaining psycho-challenges I was having and the problems they were giving me. After considering the many pluses and minuses, I maintained that I didn't need them. I wanted a certain psycho-alertness to remain within me, should I need it, but due to the issues it had caused me these last few weeks, I thought it better to let that go too and instead rely on my instinct as to how to react as the situation demanded.

What happened next was that this kind, gentle, and caring spiritual supervisor's voice said, 'Since you no longer need this part, it shall be released.' That was when I felt something exit my body, and inside me, I felt calm and relaxed.

In the early morning, I woke up and felt relieved to have this new, free sensation within me. It felt like a small burden removed. And a couple of weeks later, I hadn't considered that I might have been manipulated in any way, regardless of what had been said. When an interesting discussion is started, I remain relaxed and involved the whole time. Today, as before, I occasionally sense the first stages of my routine kicking off, and then it withers into nothing as if the subsequent stages are now missing. I can remain calm in the new situations I will have to face.

Who would have thought that cannabis would have had such a profound effect on me?

About eleven weeks after completing this fourth Sweet Spot, I noticed some erratic emotions in me. I would have sudden bouts of intense happiness, followed by deep bouts of sadness, an emotional splurge of anger, and finally by hopelessness. After that, came intermittent periods of intense laughter. My emotions had been switched on for the first time as I experienced these new feelings.

The best analogy I can think of is a fluorescent tube that erratically flickers on and off until it remains on. When it's switched on, my emotions are on, and I'm experiencing them.

Then it switches off, as do my feelings. And then another emotional fluorescent tube flickers on and off, and I live that particular emotion to the full when the tube is on.

Over time, an increasing number of different emotions start to flicker simultaneously. It is like a piece of old and unused equipment being turned on for the first time and having problems starting up. What is super is that the flickering is happening less often, and the emotions are becoming more and more consistent. A side effect is that I feel a little vulnerable as I navigate this phase.

An example of this vulnerability is that my wife and I once had an intensive discussion, which got a bit heated because I was emotionally confused at that moment. In the past, I usually felt in control of every argument I had, and whoever it was with. When it was finished, my brain continued to happily mash through that discussion further by planning and storing up points for later, should they be needed.

These points were generally seen from my point of view only. This time, after the heated debate, we discussed all the issues affecting us and found a super solution that helped us. I remained focused on the points under consideration instead of continually jumping from one perspective to the other. This is super. I have noticed a difference in my thinking over this last year, but this was another cherry on the cake for me.

Although this new two-sided discussion went well, I didn't feel in control, and there was no scheming, planning, or manipulation. I was just focused on finding a way forward with my wife. Even after the discussion and once we had found a way forward, I felt relieved that we had achieved this. We then considered how I could unilaterally help us both achieve a better solution.

There was not one manipulative thought flying through my mind at all. This is an entirely new experience for me. My newly discovered emotional response may be weak and erratic, but it is a unique experience. I am curious to see whether this continues growing within me or whether I have reached my new emotional limit.

Another example is that we love films and watch quite a few in our free time. I usually watch a film, enjoy it, and then forget it. Now, I choke up on those sad moments, get angry at a character's stupidity (yes, I know it is part of the story), and laugh at scenes I would never usually consider funny. And not only that, we're even having great discussions about the film we've just seen, and I love it.

At other times, I'm as cold as ice again (the tubes are off) and back to my emotionless self. When the emotions are working and I feel something building up that I haven't felt before, I must consider how I need to react and think. Maybe this is a mistake, and I should allow the emotion to take its natural course.

After reflection, I can say that I like this new feeling of being better able to understand my and other people's emotions, although I do need to learn how to react a little friendlier or whether I need to respond at all. I have a massive learning curve ahead of me as I gather new experience. I hope that my emotions stabilise, either on or off, or at least that I find some consistency so I can better determine how I need to be.

I have carried out the three tests again (psychopath, sociopath and narcissist). Here are the outcomes:

Psychopath test: My first result before the fourth Sweet Spot was 29/40, then 8/40 one day after the fourth Sweet Spot. A month later, it increased to 12/40. And now, two months after completing the fourth Sweet Spot, it is 5/40. I believe the most significant change occurred after I took the cannabis biscuits to help me sleep and met my spiritual supervisor. As I've mentioned before, since then, I have started experiencing mixed emotions and have gained a better understanding of others' perspectives.

Narcissist test: My first result before the fourth Sweet Spot was 31/40, then 4/40 one day after the fourth Sweet Spot. A month later, it increased to 5/40. And now, two months after completing the fourth Sweet Spot, it is 5/40. It is wonderful to see that the result has stabilised. I notice my old narcissistic tendencies are no longer there, and this result confirms that.

Sociopath test: My first result before the fourth Sweet Spot was 20/25, then 6/25 one day after the fourth Sweet Spot. A month later, it dropped to 5/25. And now it has stabilised at 6/25. Drifting between one or two points is fine, and according to this test, I am no longer a sociopath. I hope this remains true.

I know and appreciate that these tests are from the internet and are not done by a specialist. I have had to be honest with myself to get the correct results. Yet, the changes I notice reflect the results I have scored. I see an emotional difference in me, and it is my emotions that have just woken up after a long, long time of being dormant and are now stabilising.

Now my mind is calmer and my physical body is more relaxed throughout the day. I feel mentally free from the bounds I have carried around all my life. I understand that it is impossible to determine the permanency of these changes after only two months, and I know I will have to monitor my progress over the following months and years.

If this is the case with me, let's consider the help psychedelics could offer to millions and millions of people out there who are enclosed in their restrictive world and not living the lives they should. Is it fair to leave all these people to suffer for the rest of their lives when it could be avoided?

We know psychedelics help against autism, alcoholism, Alzheimer's, and numerous other mental and physical issues, so why not against extreme psychopathy, sociopathy and narcissism? The benefits this would provide for humankind would be immeasurable. I hope one day we will find out, and if this is indeed the case, that psychedelics are put to work where they are genuinely needed.

And what about military personnel? Soldiers who have gone through traumatic and stressful situations could undergo a 24-hour treatment programme with psychedelics and could be mentally fit for active service virtually the next day or two, instead of layering one military trauma on top of the other for them to deal with once they have left the forces.

A great idea, maybe, but we know from experience that no government protects its (ex-)personnel's mental health. If they did, we wouldn't be having as many suicides and ongoing PTSD cases as we currently do.

After eleven weeks of completing the fourth Sweet Spot, it's time to take stock. Let's consider the area of health, fitness, and sport.

Since completing the fourth Sweet Spot, I have been doing the *Insanity* DVD course daily. I have commented earlier on my experiences of this over the first four weeks, including the beginning of the 1-week recovery sessions. The second part of *Insanity* has been a real challenge. Adding an extra round of exercises shown on each DVD means completing each round takes nearly an hour.

Over the past four weeks, I have always been exhausted at the end of each session, as the intensity is high. Although micro-dosing helps, my lack of overall fitness plays a significant role in my struggle, and then there's the imbalance with my legs that I must constantly watch.

But on Day 54 of *Insanity,* I noticed two things. Firstly, I had more energy to invest in the routines and completed more exercises than usual before collapsing in a pool of sweat. A significant improvement physically. The second is that my right leg appears to have noticeably strengthened.

Today is the last day of *Insanity,* and these last four weeks have been very challenging. I have completed every session, except for one. I officially missed one day in the recovery week due to a slight fever. I had missed two sessions, one after another, but I used my rest day to make up for the day I was ill and trained on the rest day at the end of the week. Regarding the last four weeks of Insanity, I didn't manage the Cardio Abs training part because I was too exhausted to complete it.

The best news over this short time frame is that I have lost 11kg. At one point, my weight stabilised for about a week before continuing to drop. The reason for this weight stabilisation was that we have just had Christmas, New Year and various gatherings with friends and family.

I didn't eat much more over this short period, but I had been testing different foods, including some sweets, to determine whether I had control over the dietary issues. And it appears I have. As I have said before, I had a pig-out day in the first few weeks after completing the fourth Sweet Spot, and the next day, I had it under control again.

Now that the holidays are over, I have my dietary control in hand, and it's a significant improvement over the situation before my last therapy session. I still need to lose another 9kg to reach my ideal weight, but realistically, I would be pleased to lose another 6kg by the end of this year.

What's Next?
Hmm, this is an interesting question that quickly answered itself. This revelation came as I was finishing the final stages of this book, ready for print (again), when I had the urge to carry out a fifth Sweet Spot therapeutic session. The outcome of this session blew me away to such an extent that, at first, I didn't

know how to respond, as I am sure what I am about to describe may be a problem for some people.

Because of the intensity of my experience, I even considered leaving it out altogether. However, several friends who have helped me through this experiment commented that this last session is essential to my continual development, and it should be included as it brings closure to this part of my life's journey.

Sweet Spot No 5 – The Master Reset

We shall not cease from exploration
And the end of all our exploring
Will be to arrive where we started
And know the place for the first time
                                    The Four Quartets, **T.S. *Eliot***

This fifth Sweet Spot session brought my experiments to a perfect close. It was, however, the hardest to write up as it took me way beyond my most profound beliefs and expectations. What I have gone through in the previous four Sweet Spots has helped me find my true self and deal with my past, enabling me to live a new life free from those previous burdens.

But all those experiences that I have gone through this last year pale insignificantly compared to what I have just experienced with this fifth one. Who would have expected something like this could have happened to me?

But before we begin, please keep in mind that what I am about to describe is my experience as I currently understand it, with minimal knowledge on the subject, even though I am still processing and coming to terms with it. Another point I want to mention is that I have left a lot out of what I have just experienced, as I feel it is too controversial and offensive to some. Nevertheless, I hope you enjoy reading this thought-provoking experience as much as I have participating in it.

However, I want to bring two points to your attention before proceeding. Firstly, I have had an almost lifelong problem and dislike regarding religion, the church in all its different flavours and the confusing roles they play in society. For me, in a nutshell, it has become such a complicated and unnecessarily meta-physical dance that has grown into an excessive and expensive misrepresentation of God's name to control, manipulate and in many cases terrify the masses for its ends. The second point is that for the whole of my life, I have thought that there is no God in any shape or form and that we are alone in this world and in this Universe.

To help me explain the first stages of this life-changing experience that I have just gone through and how it has affected me, I would like to simplify the description as much as possible, not only in explaining this to you, but to help me on my path in understanding it. For these next few minutes, I will disregard all written 'religious' texts that include those impressive collections of opinions from either a single male or a group of men, which have been collated over the years since we've been able to record our thoughts.

Whether these opinions are accurate isn't the point, and I prefer to leave that discussion for theologians and those who are more qualified. I also want to disregard individual religious groups, whether Christian, Jewish, Muslim, etc., as well as liturgy-prayer, routines, stories, and saints of the modern era.

In other words, I want to take us back to the basics, back to the very early days thousands of years ago, when all we had was one of the first Shamans wanting to talk to God about a problem. This Shaman had some issue, whether it be concerning illness, conflict, crops, livestock, etc, such that they took a psychedelic of some sort, depending on where they were in the world. And this is what I want to categorise as 'religion' in its purest form.

As civilisation and knowledge grew, so did its routines and rituals, which began to develop and have become more complicated and esoteric. Shamans isolated themselves more over time, and several intelligent thinkers have created various drawings, texts, and opinions to provide a 'guide' to a way of thinking. But the more we write and draw, the more confusing the simple message becomes: maybe God is easier to approach than with thought.

Here we have God, billions, if not trillions, of years old, who outstrips all our planetary life and the life span of all religions put together. God has created the building blocks with finite combinations and the Universal laws for us to follow. We make up only a tiny fraction of God's whole Universal programme on this planet.

We know that the church destroyed many pagan rituals, so we have sadly lost so many roots of our spiritual history. However, the early church continued to use and adapt many of the same pagan rituals by rebranding them as their own, so all is not entirely lost. Fortunately, through this activity, it looks like the Church has preserved the very basic and fundamental principle of the Shaman, and that is how to reach God through the use of psychedelics.

I'm sure there are many other sources still available worldwide that we could tap into to understand how to reach God. Still, I would like to stick with the European church and its history for ease of explanation, as many of us have some understanding of it.

However, the inspiring drawings in the impressive *Canterbury Psalter* contain a beautiful Shamanic guide for us to follow (should we wish). Looking carefully at this stunningly decorated book, we can see psychedelic mushrooms in several beautifully decorated old pictures.

I want to add here as a side-note that there are other lovely preserved sources depicting the use of psychedelics in old churches within Europe that were probably used as guides by early Christian Shamans to help contact God. Many religious experts deny this, but which of them have tested this thesis out to determine whether it could be the case?

Maybe the only way to find out what these drawings mean is to 'partake in God's flesh' by eating some of the divine mushroom, otherwise known for the last thousand years as the 'little Saints', or to 'drink God's blood' made of a fresh or recycled mushroom juice/tea.

It seems pretty possible that, whereas these drawings show us how we may approach God individually, many people cannot see these clues in their normal state. By partaking in a psychedelic, the drawings may speak to us through imagery and even guide us in finding the answers we seek.

Before I make myself sound even crazier than I am, I think this is a good time to describe my fifth Sweet Spot experience, and then continue to explain what effect this has had on me. From what I have written, you may already have a good idea. So, here goes…

As I start this session, I ask myself whether I can recognise and understand any remaining internal blocking points I am still unaware of, so I can undertake a 'Master Reset' of my past life. And as I ask myself this, it is by pure chance that I have the *Canterbury Psalter* open on my computer.

I have just finished reading the fantastic book, *The Psychedelic Gospels,* by Jerry and Julie Brown, about the possible use of psychedelics in religion to help us come into contact with God, and I am in the middle of reviewing some of their references to help develop my own opinion about their research.

As the session gets underway, I notice the effects of the mushrooms, and I feel attracted towards the computer. And as

I look at those beautiful pictures within the *Canterbury Psalter*, they come alive, and some start to merge, eventually producing a new image with some depth and detail. The best way to describe this is to use a more complicated version of those 'Magic Eye' images that appear when the eyes are relaxed enough to see a simple 3-D shape, word, or phrase on some normally unrecognisable jagged picture.

Dancing around this new image are several words from the surrounding text that create new sentences before my eyes, but alas, I don't pay enough attention to them to recognise what is written. Although I can't understand Latin, there is some intuitive comprehension within me regarding the meaning of these sentences, when suddenly, as if by magic, a portal-gate opens up before me.

It might be hard for you to believe what I have just said here when such an experience hasn't been lived through. Believe me, I'm still trying to get my head around it myself. Suddenly, I feel as though I am pulled into this new moving 3-D image, travel through a portal, and before I know it, I am in front of this powerful energy.

Yes, I know, all my life I have said there is no God, and now I know how wrong I have been. But this genderless energy is not as we perceive God to be in the forms described or painted over the centuries. This constantly moving force of energy has some element of similarity to our documented experiences, but doesn't appear to be a human form, except that it reminds me of an undefinable figure form postured on clouds with the vast Universe behind it, but that's the only similarity I can recognise.

I could use only one abstract noun to describe this energy's aura and presence: the word 'love'. This energy emanates unconditional love, caring, and devotion as if there were no tomorrow, regardless of our history, just like our mother, favourite auntie, or grandma does when we need them the most.

Being bathed and wrapped up in her incredible, reassuring, protective, and radiating love is something I will never forget. Looking around me, I see that we are connected, and we (my spirit and its energy) are smaller than the smallest Universal building blocks it creates. These blocks are the base of everything in life and the Universe itself. Yet, when I look closer, I see that each of those building blocks appears to be a Universe within itself with its own God (or force of energy), spiritually connected to ours.

Even though it, in its single entity, is smaller than the smallest thing that can be conceivably thought within our Universe, it, as a whole, is the purest form of a life force that binds the fundamental particles together. It makes the proton bond with the constructed neutron and accurately drives the constructed electron to fly around this core. Its spirit binds one atom to the other, continuing to bind everything to the very boundaries of our Universe.

As I look around, we are all like pins rising from her universal energy, providing us with this Universal connection to everything around us. Only when a defined combination arises with the building block and its energy do we gain a living consciousness, such that this independent energy gives us physical life and independent thought.

A way to describe this energy is like spiritual mycelium that spreads unseen through an infinite network, circulates through our planet, and links us to all creatures, plants, and trees as One. For all the creatures that live in this Universe, our subconscious is a part of our soul.

Just as I have theorised that our finite Universe is a proton, neutron or an electron, depending on the Universe's potential charge, that we may well be forming an atom from another parallel Universe with its own God. And all those parallel Universes forming atoms are held together by a higher or greater God or a higher energy within that higher Universe. And what if we take this concept further, how do we know when to stop?

Okay, that's enough. Even I'm starting to scare myself with these new thoughts. Although I find this new subject and perspective of our Universe and its connection to life, how long will my thoughts continue to expand on this experience and understanding I have just gone through?

I've mentioned that this genderless energy, many like to call 'God', leaves me feeling obliged to humanise and personify it, but under a different name, 'Soma'. When humanised, Soma can only be a she, maybe because it is the creator of all the interlocking parts of all living species and inert materials surrounding us. Indeed, who else could create and give birth to such beauty and life in this Universe than a woman with such a minute and powerful finite amount of building blocks?

Those blocks have followed the Universal laws to create the elements we know today (and maybe some remain unknown to us). But could there be several Creators? We have the caretaker of this Universe, God or Soma (the Spiritual), the father, and the second, who I now recognise as the creator of physical Life, is our mother.

Regardless of our relationship with the latter or what she has gone through, I now see her as God's true representative. There can be no greater Gods to respect and admire than those who can give birth to life. We as men can help initiate that magical process, but it's women who have the power to continue to create and bring this amazing cycle to a close.

So, where does that leave us men who have taken the initiative to write so many texts over all of these years and who have been the cause of so much death and destruction in the name of God?

Although we (both sexes) work and live as a unit in all aspects of everyday life, men are both the other part of women within a unified team and their protector, and I think rightly so. Men and the community are crucial at those key moments so that women can give birth to a stable cycle of life for our future generations within a safe and stable environment. We are unique, and what we are missing within ourselves, we find in the other.

Back to the subject of communicating directly with God through psychedelics. In my opinion, this is all we need to be in touch with this powerful energy we call God, Soma, or whatever you want.

The rest is just pomp and circumstance, dressage, an act, or a mass tool used to describe it to manipulate and control the masses so they behave in a certain way. Wouldn't it be better for each of us who wants to be able to find out and define it as it is within our inner eye or perspective? Or is it better to have it as an absent friend and to idolise it?

I'm not saying it's wrong, I'm just asking which is preferable. Yet, if we want to put this hard-working force on a pedestal and it helps someone to get on with life or deal with difficult situations, that is fine. If someone needs to lop off a piece of skin, for example, from someone else or encourage others to partake in some other initiation ceremony to join a religious clan, and that helps them, that's great if both are in agreement.

And if someone wants to believe in the resurrection of Jesus or that he fled to France with his wife, Madelene, after the crucifixion, or to have an instrument of his torture hanging somewhere in the house, or that it helps to have pictures of (human) saints hanging on the wall, then go for it. Ultimately, it's your life, beliefs, and choices, just like I have to decide what I need. And I am now re-defining what I believed for all these years.

At the start of this session, I did not know that God, Soma or the Universe would be responsible for the proper Master Reset of my life. Nothing was asked, and nothing was spoken, yet there was an understanding between the two of us when it happened. This Master Reset she gave me has resolved any final issues that I was unaware of. It felt like a huge burden I didn't know I still had that was suddenly removed. What a relief this is to me.

What now? Does that mean I'm now a re-born convert who will start going to church to pray and ask for forgiveness for my previous sins?

Although right at the beginning of this therapeutic Sweet Spot session, I experienced my (re-)birth, for me, the answer is a definite 'no'. Why? Because from my new experience, that's not how it seems to work. If it, Soma, can create the spiritual and physical fundamental blocks of this Universe, right up to (and more) creating living forms, the strength and support of both male and female to support and protect each other within a community, such that each of our mothers can freely create us, nurture us and to give birth to our life. Then I can make a life of my own in their honour by providing a foundation for future generations to rely on.

Suppose I get stuck again, which can happen to us all at some point, I now know how to ask for her help with the use of psychedelics and without having to join that mass of white noise along with millions of others who are hoping for some form of recognition for the answer to their prayers. Whether I need the aid of the *Canterbury Psalter* again, I doubt it; only time will tell. I guess it's only one source of help among many available to us, since we have been contacting and talking with God, Soma or the Universe for millions of years.

This experience has been a significant life-changing and an amazing spiritual experience for me. Please remember that what I have noted above is my interpretation of what I have just gone through. I know I have written it a bit clumsily and crudely as this new way of thinking is still forming in my mind, so I ask for your patience and understanding.

And if we wish, we can also realise we have the option through the resources and guides of the little saints or other psychedelics to help us make our way to it (or towards our inner selves). Again, the rest is up to you whether you agree with my opinion. And if you don't, that's fine, please respect it, as I do with yours. Even if I turn out to be wrong, it doesn't matter if it is a necessary stepping stone to help me get to the next level of understanding.

Summary of Events

Overall, while writing this, I'm so at peace with myself. I thought the fourth Sweet Spot was the ultimate experience in releasing me from my past and enhancing my way on my life journey. However, the effects of this fifth session continue to exceed all expectations daily. Here is a weekly breakdown of what I have gone through.

One Week Later...

To begin with, I was in a daze and felt a little confused about life and what I had gone through. I had a 'funny head' for about four days. It wasn't a headache or a migraine, but I felt like changes were happening inside me, affecting my way of thinking. Perhaps this was down to a rewiring of the neurons in my brain.

Things that were once important to me were becoming less so. An example of this is material wealth. I look around our apartment and wonder why I ever bought that? Time to get rid of it. My previous attitude would have been, 'I've got to have that, because...' followed by a relatively weak reason and then bought it. This attitude has gone.

Two Weeks Later...

It was this week that I hit a bit of a downer, felt dizzy and continued to struggle with some headaches. Perhaps this was a symptom of creating new neuro-circuits and shutting down older, restrictive ones. Who needs ECT treatment when we have the power of psychedelics?

Charlie participates in an experiment in one of my favourite books, *Flowers for Algernon* by Daniel Keyes. As he experiences intellectual and mental changes, he starts to re-interpret his relationship with his 'friends' and the world around him in a completely different light. I am in a similar situation and realise how much of my life I have been fighting in vain against practically everything.

There is no fight in me anymore. Instead, there are several clear paths ahead that have always been there, but it is only now that I can see them. Many of these wonderful paths are now overgrown and no longer passable due to my age, and that hurts, yet there are still some interesting options to consider. Which path I need to take is still a little unclear; maybe the key lies in the writing of this book or something else I haven't yet discovered. Only time will tell...

Three weeks later...

I've still been getting those occasional 'headaches' that are different to other ones I have previously had. Then one day, something dramatic happened. It was like a 'click' in my brain, and the pain stopped. It was literally like a bright light had been switched on.

Suddenly, everything looked brighter, rosier, and my energy levels shot through the roof. This led to me feeling happier, more contented, and far more productive without any self-doubt creeping in. For example, I still have concerns about the content of this fifth Sweet Spot I have written. However, the self-doubts I would have had previously are no longer there. I can assess this decision of mine, whether to include this experience in this book, more objectively.

Also, I have carried out the three tests again regarding being a psychopath, sociopath and narcissist. Here are the results:

Psychopath test: My first result before starting the fourth Sweet Spot was 29/40; one day after the fourth Sweet Spot, it dropped to 8/40. A month later, it had increased to 12/40. Two months after completing the fourth Sweet Spot, it dropped to 5/50. This, I put down to the effects of the cannabis biscuits when I met my spiritual supervisor, thus eliminating all of my psycho-voice. Three weeks after completing the fifth Sweet Spot, the result is 4/40, and I still have no psycho-voice in my head, and I can still focus easily on the present and my surroundings.

Narcissist test: My first result before starting the fourth Sweet Spot was 31/40; one day after the fourth Sweet Spot, it dropped to 4/40. A month later, it increased to 5/40, which made me unconcerned. Two months after completing the fourth Sweet Spot, it stabilised at 5/40. Three weeks after completing the fifth Sweet Spot, it has fallen to 2/40. It is excellent that it is so surprisingly low, and that confirms that I no longer have any narcissistic tendencies.

Sociopath test: My first result before starting the fourth Sweet Spot was 20/25, but one day after the fourth Sweet Spot, it dropped to 6/25. A month later, it dropped another point to 5/25, which gives me no concerns. Two months later, it increased slightly to 6/25, and I am okay with this. Three weeks after completing the fifth Sweet Spot, the result stabilised at 6/25, and I am pleased about this. I am no longer a sociopath.

Four weeks later...

This has been a bit of a weird week for me. I've been having several daily flashbacks, and they are different from the ones I have had previously. Out of nowhere, I see scenes of myself where I am observing myself and how isolated, confused and alone I was. These flashbacks happen randomly with no trigger, or at least none I can recognise.

I may be at home, walking down the street, or working on something, and then 'poof' I have this recollection. For most of the week, I have experienced flashbacks from my early childhood before I was a teenager. However, I'm now having flashbacks from my teenage years to adulthood, and it is showing me how isolated I was from everything around me, even in my older years.

It has prompted a question about how I was perceived as a child, a teenager, and an adult. Unfortunately, Mum is no longer here, so I asked my sister. This discussion was a revelation; she gave me some things to consider. What was said in the conversation isn't appropriate for this book. Sorry. However, it has given me other avenues to think about and is helping me to understand myself a lot better.

Five weeks later...

Like my experiences with the fifth Sweet Spot, I have also considered leaving this section out. I'm at the absolute limit of understanding what I am going through, and I am a little worried that it will be misconstrued somehow. After some discussions with my wife, I was convinced that including this is a good idea as it provides a complete picture of what is happening to me.

I was thinking about what I have achieved in life, and I realised that all we have is borrowed from the Universe. Ultimately, nothing is ours and nothing belongs to us during our real (physical) time on this planet. Whether it be a pair of shoes, a car, a television, a house, money, love, happiness, pain, etc, it's all on loan.

At some point, we give it back to the Universe to be recycled for reuse. That's fine, you may say, but my next thought was that the Universe has given us billions of years for a life cycle, such that the Universe can easily break down those no-longer-needed tools and remains, which is fine.

When we create and use a tool (product) that is no longer needed and can't be recycled, are we disrespecting the laws of the Universe and not respecting the ultimate damage that could be caused to our future generations? My other question is what will happen to us over a more extended period when we continue not to fit in with the Universal Laws?

And taking this thought one step further, what is our role in life? Maybe she has chosen us all as the planet's caretakers and other living creatures. Doing this ensures a cyclic balance in all aspects of life and death.

Not only that, but maybe we are also being tested on how we handle and use these finite Universal building block combinations responsibly. For example, specific chains of building blocks can cause irreparable death and damage if used. And maybe this is our ultimate test of responsibility as joint caretakers on this tiny planet for our future.

But what if this irresponsible damage we are doing as human beings is her cancer? As long as we are contained on this planet doing our ills, then her cancer is contained. Only once we can inhabit another planet, reaching further distant planets becomes much easier, so the disease spreads.

At this point, we can't control who will ultimately leave this planet. As her cancer spreads, her Universal force weakens, just as it does with us. And then what? Will our Universe implode on itself, or will it have a knock-on effect on the other Universes alongside us and above us and thus ultimately destroy the lower Universes that are entirely reliant on us for their survival?

Does this make me crazy or highlight something I'm still trying to comprehend? I'm not sure myself. Now that this book is complete, I intend to investigate this further. Hmm, where do I start with such a subject?

Six to Nine Weeks Later...

I want to group these three weeks because the major transition is ending. As each day passes, I feel calmer, more self-assured, and more relaxed. The flashbacks come less often, leaving me with more internal peace, and my mind opens up to new thoughts and considerations. When the flashbacks do come back, they confirm some small minor issue I can easily let go of.

All my headaches have disappeared, and I have clarity in my thoughts throughout the day. I sleep wonderfully, and all my Dark Thoughts are gone. The remaining tension in my chest has been released, and I can breathe easier.

A rather significant issue I have had for many years is that I have had a toxic 'friend' that I have not been able to deal with. She reminds me too much of how I was before starting this experiment, and that unsettles me quite a bit. It's a one-way relationship that exhausts me from being in his company.

In my psychopathic days, I always felt I was playing my strategies against his, and that was exhausting for me. Now I feel vulnerable, exhausting me, trying to find new ways to protect myself. After considering this relationship for a few days and upon reflection, I've come to realise that I need to do the same for her, given how my close friends have accepted me and my exhaustive ways.

This thought has turned my perspective around, and I have more acceptance, patience and understanding for her. And by going through this new thought process, I can recognise and accept how much pain I was suffering under and how much of a burden I was putting upon others. Not only do I feel this newfound freedom within me in a different way, but I now understand how toxic I was to other people. I can only apologise for what I have done to those who have suffered because of me. However, I don't think I can apologise for what I was, without knowing enough of myself to know what torment I was going through against myself.

Eight to Twelve Weeks Later...

Before I explain what is happening to me here, I'm asking myself how many cherries on the cake I can have. What is happening now, and I'm only focusing on one point, is one of my last wishes coming true: my weight is dropping again without any active intervention.

Earlier, I mentioned that I wanted to reach 70kg by the end of the year and would be happy if I reach a stable 75kg by the end of the year, as this would take me from 'low' risk to 'very low/no' risk of a heart attack for my age group. In these four weeks, I have just passed my 75kg marker.

But what am I doing differently? I can say I am letting my body decide what it needs and am supporting it. I'm not eating less, just differently. My carb intake has seriously dropped, as has my high-fat intake (and there's nothing more delicious than fat and sugary carbs mixed). I'm separating the two when I eat them and balancing out what makes me feel good, rather than a feeling of contentedness.

I still have another seven months before the end of the year and am curious whether I can reach my goal weight or whether it will level out once again before reaching it. This change in my diet feels like supporting my inner feelings and thoughts. That famous phrase, 'you are what you eat', has some value. However, based on my understanding, I think it is more appropriate to rearrange it slightly to say 'you eat what you are', which has more meaning.

In summary, this weight loss is telling me I have removed my emotional baggage, dealt with my history and my inner torment. Regardless of what anybody thinks about my thoughts and experiences, as documented in this book, I can categorically say that I am finally free.

The End

Do not believe in something because it is reported. Do not believe in something because generations have practised it or made it a tradition or part of a culture. Do not believe in something because a scripture says it is so. Do not believe in something believing a god has inspired it. Do not believe in something a teacher tells you to. Do not believe in something because the authorities say it is so. Do not believe in hearsay, rumour, speculative opinion, public opinion, or mere acceptance of logic and inference alone. Help yourself, accept as entirely accurate only that which is praised by the wise and which you test for yourself and know to be good for yourself and others.

The Kalama Sutta, **Buddha**

When I first started this micro-dosing experiment, I never, even for one moment, considered I would be able to take it this far and remove all traces of my PTSD, anxiety, depression, and other restrictive issues entirely, let alone have such a profound spiritual experience I have just described in the last chapter. I thought maybe my problems would be softened a little and that I could live with them a bit better with micro-dosing.

I never thought I would be able to join society again and feel a part of it, yet here I am doing just that. And I never thought I could be as relaxed and focused as I am now. Psychedelics have changed my mindset completely, especially with the removal of the psychopath, sociopath and narcissist within me, such that this has enabled me to deal with many new and sometimes more complex issues in a relaxed and controlled manner. And most of all, I never thought I would experience Soma and the Universe the way I have.

However, focusing on the problems I had, a question I still cannot answer is whether dealing with the psychopath in me was the right way forward in releasing those lifelong problems. Could I have managed all of what I have gone through without an NLP Breakthrough session, or would it have been too much for me emotionally if I had tried to tackle it all at once? Would a single and ultimate Master Reset Sweet Spot session have triggered other mental concerns, or would they have been eliminated? Or was it better, as in this case, to work through each of my inner layers until I managed to destroy my problems in differing stages? Should someone know or have an inkling, please let me know.

So, to re-review a question I have asked before, do I think that psychedelics should be available to all?

I believe a proportion of the population would be able to use psychedelics sensibly to help themselves cope with varying issues, as well as for pure enjoyment. However, from my experience after the fourth session, I firmly believe it's not a good idea to do a therapy session alone, especially when working on some seriously intense issues.

There are millions of people spread across this planet who suffer from PTSD due to some abuse or trauma, and I think that prescription medication cannot always provide a satisfactory solution in either the short- or long-term. They may help to hide the pain for a while, but in the long run, it's not enough. We need to get to the root of the problem as quickly and as effectively as possible, and I think psychedelics are one of the only real options we have.

I think I have only scratched the surface of their potential in this book. The sooner psychedelics are made legal, the better the chance we have to reverse the current trend of ever-increasing mental and other stress-related issues that many are struggling to cope with.

With psychedelics, it's not just about getting high, as many lawmakers like to think, it's about getting help to seek solutions to our problems, and I think we should all have the personal right to select and use what we believe best for our psyche.

My experiences to date, both with micro-dosing as well as with therapeutic dosing, have been unwittingly and perfectly geared to this end. At the moment, I have had no urge to use psychedelics for purely recreational purposes as I still have a lot to process and understand from my last Sweet Spot session, but that doesn't mean I wouldn't try it sometime in the future.

One thing some people talk about who have taken psychedelics for therapy is that it's like hitting a Master Reset on their life's issues, as with my fifth Sweet Spot therapeutic session confirmed for me. I am not sure that some of us may have different reset 'buttons' for other issues, and some may have just the one. I know that within my first Sweet Spot, I hit some reset regarding Mum and my guilt and shame and the acceptance of death.

Regarding the second and third Sweet Spot, although I have gone through changes and have learnt a lot from them, I'm not sure I would say any reset happened. What I would say is that I have had several 'aha' moments, points of realisation about my eating, how I unwittingly dissociated myself from life, and about no longer wanting to be here on this planet.

I understood how my lack of self-confidence and self-respect had turned me into the bitter recluse I had become. The fourth Sweet Spot hit another major reset button that released me from the previous burdens I had become aware of, but I don't think it reset everything.

It was this fifth Sweet Spot session, however, that has reset pretty much everything else. How long this will last, time will tell. Maybe I will need to do a top-up once a year to keep this Master Reset at its optimum, and if that's the case, I can happily live with that. Suddenly, the future I have ahead of me now looks more assured, more than ever before.

What more could one ask for?

Closure

The mushrooms have been consumed, and I no longer need them, not even for micro-dosing. To you, my reader, it's time for me to say goodbye and thank you for being with me on this, a significant part of my life journey. You have shared the challenges I have faced and observed how these have changed me. You have seen how each of us has the potential to be what we deserve to be, regardless of whether we have suffered trauma or not.

One last point has become apparent to me: the answers we are searching for to our problems aren't found in books, food, medication, alcohol, or other hard drugs, although they may give us some short-term relief. The solution lies within us, and we owe it to ourselves to identify and work through these problems using the most appropriate tools for our health and sanity.

I once remember reading a quote many years ago from David Bowie that I had never understood, until now: *Religion is for people who fear hell, spirituality is for people who have been there.* I feel I understand this so clearly now that I have left that place of darkness. I can breathe freely for the first time in my life, and I am welcomed into the Universe with open arms that have long been awaiting my return. All this is the real recognition that my new physical and spiritual journey is just beginning...

Possible Uses and Benefits of Psychedelics

It is dangerous to be right when the government is wrong.

Voltaire

Here is an alphabetical list of potential medicinal/non-medicinal uses with cannabis, MDMA, LSD, Ayahuasca, Ibogaine and magic mushrooms:

Acne, addiction, aging, alcoholism, Alzheimer's, ankylosing spondylitis, anorexia nervosa, antibiotic, anti-inflammatory, antifungal, antiemetic, anti-depressive, anxiety, (nausea and vomiting), appetite stimulation, amyotrophic lateral sclerosis (ALS), arthritis, asthma, atherosclerosis, ADD, ADHD, autism, autoimmune, brainwave improvement, cachexia (wasting syndrome), cancer, cancer pain, cerebral palsy, chemo induced nausea and vomiting, chronic pain, chronic obstructive pulmonary disease, cluster headache, creativity boost, crime reduction, Crohn's disease, cystic fibrosis, dermatitis, diabetes (type I and II), depression, dystonia, eczema, emotional empathy, endometriosis, epilepsy, fertility, fibromyalgia, fracture, gastrointestinal disorders, glaucoma, head trauma, helplessness, herpes, hepatitis, hiccups, HIV/AIDS, Huntington's disease, hypertension, improved quality of life, injury, inflammation, insomnia, child labour pains, lupus, migraine, Meige syndrome, metabolic syndrome, mental disorders, menstrual cramps, mood disorders, motion sickness, multiple sclerosis, muscle spasms, muscular dystrophy, neuropathy, neuroprotective antioxidant, non-organic failure to thrive in new-borns, obesity, OCD, osteoarthritis, osteoporosis, pain, paraplegia, parasite removal, Parkinson's, Pharmaceutical alternatives, premenstrual syndrome, pruritus, quadriplegia, promotion of pro-social behaviours, pruritis, PTSD, PMS, psoriasis, rejection reduction of transplanted organs, rheumatism, schizophrenia, scleroderma, sexual dysfunction, sickle cell, sleep apnoea, spasticity, spinal cord injury, split personality, stress, stroke, Tourette's, therapy aide, traumatic brain injury, Wilson's.

As scientific research into psychedelics progresses, so does the list.

For those who wish to read more about how cannabis can help against certain illnesses, I can recommend *Marihuana, The Forbidden Medicine* by Lester Grinspoon and James Bakalar.

References and Further Reading

Researching, understanding and expanding my knowledge on psychedelics and other legal and illegal drugs, this material comes primarily through the books of respected scientists and authors on these subjects.

I have occasionally used websites as my primary source (NHS, for example) when I thought it appropriate to help me verify this material or to gather a more comprehensive understanding of specific subjects. I must be clear about my investigative approach here, as I am neither a doctor nor a scientist.

Below, I have listed (in no particular order) everything I have used for this book and plenty of other material for further reading should there be an interest. In certain sections of this book, I have given my opinion. However, that should be clear to the reader when I have done this.

Books and Weblinks

Books Used on Drugs and Psychedelics:
Dr Richard Louis Miller: *Psychedelic Medicine: The Healing Powers of LSD, MDMA, Psilocybin and Ayahuasca*
Aldous Huxley: *The Doors of Perception*
James Fadiman: *The Psychedelics Explorer's Guide*
Ayelet Waldman: *A Really Good Day*
David Nutt: *Drugs: Without The Hot Air*
Paula Mallea: *The War On Drugs: A Failed Experiment*
Timothy Leary: *The Psychedelic Experience*
Mark Flaherty: *Shedding the Layers*
Jay Stevens: *Storming Heaven: LSD And The American Dream*
Stanislav Grof and Christina Grof: *Holotropic Breathwork*
Stanislav Grof: *Realms of the Human Unconsciousness*
Alexander and Ann Shulgin: *Pihkal and Tihkal*

Dr Richard Louis Miller: *Psychedelic Medicine*
Sir Richard Branson: *Ending the War on Drugs*
Max Daly & Steve Sampson: *Narcomania*
Tom Shroder: *Acid Test*
Jerry & Julie Brown: *The Psychedelic Gospels*
Richard Branson: *Ending the War on Drugs*
Michael Pollan: *How to Change Your Mind*
Misha Glenny: *McMafia*
Arthur Janov: *The New Primal Scream*

Cannabis as Medicine:
Lester Grinspoon and James Makalar: *Marihuana, The Forbidden Medicine*

Doctors Coming Clean
Robert S Mendelsohn: *Confessions of a Medical Heretic*
Peter Rost: *The Whistleblower*

Pharma Industry and Diet
Ben Goldacre: *Bad Pharma*
Barry Groves: *Trick and Treat*

Anslinger and the Effects of Prohibition
Johann Hari: *Chasing the Scream*

Depression
Johann Hari: *Lost Connections*

Psychopathy, Sociopathy and Narcissism
Kevin Dutton: *The Wisdom of Psychopaths*
Martha Stout: *The Sociopath Next Door*
Paul Babiak & Robert Hare: *Snakes in Suits*
Craig Malkin: *Rethinking Narcissism*
Kevin Dutton & Andy McNabb: *The Good Psychopath's Guide to Success*
James Fallon: *The Psychopath Inside*

Insanity and Schizophrenia
Nellie Bly: *Ten Days in a Mad-House*
Robert Whitaker: *Mad In America*
Robert Whitaker: *Anatomy of an Epidemic*

PTSD
Karl Smith: *There is No 'D' in PTSD*
Pete Walker: *Complex PTSD*
Rachael Keogh: *Dying to Survive*
Mark Johnson: *Wasted*

Wim Hof Method
Wim Hof: *The Way of the Iceman*

Growing Mushrooms:
L. G. Nicholas and Kerry Ogame: *Psilocybin – Mushroom Handbook – Easy Indoor and Outdoor Cultivation.*
Mandrake Ph.D., Dr K, et al.: *The Psilocybin Mushroom Bible: The Definitive Guide to Growing and Using Magic Mushrooms*

Buying Mushrooms:
Joanne Hillyer: *Psilocybin – Magic Mushrooms for the Mind*
Tom Williams: *A Quick Guide to Microdosing Psychedelics*
Frank Luft: *Microdosing LSD*

OCD:
https://iocdf.org/about-ocd/
https://tonic.vice.com/en_us/article/vbxey8/can-you-treat-ocd-with-shrooms-psychedelics
http://www.maps.org/research-archive/psilo/azproto.html
https://thethirdwave.co/psychedelics-ocd/
https://psychedelictimes.com/tag/ocd/

Autism:
https://www.autismspeaks.org/what-autism

https://www.autism.org.uk/about/what-is.aspx
https://thethirdwave.co/psychedelics-autism/
https://www.thecut.com/2016/12/psilocybin-research-looks-very-exciting.html
http://www.psychedelic-library.org/autism.htm
https://www.reddit.com/r/microdosing/comments/8hfsce/amazing_lsd_autism_microdosing/
https://www.reddit.com/r/microdosing/comments/a0xdgz/anyone_else_becoming_autistic/
https://www.reddit.com/r/microdosing/comments/58a3x8/microdosing_as_a_treatment_for_autism_spectrum/

Asperger's:
https://www.autism.org.uk/about/what-is/asperger.aspx
https://www.autismspeaks.org/what-asperger-syndrome
http://diodebridge.net/2017/05/magic-mushrooms-psilocybin-and-aspergers-syndrome-life-changing/
https://www.reddit.com/r/Drugs/comments/g773c/aspergers_and_psychedelics/
https://www.reddit.com/r/aspergers/comments/7uz4yf/nsfw_have_anyone_microdosed_lsd/
https://www.reddit.com/r/aspergers/comments/5heyz7/microdosing_lsd_for_aspergersautism/
https://thethirdwave.co/psychedelics-autism/

Tourette's:
https://tourette.org/about-tourette/overview/what-is-tourette/
https://www.reddit.com/r/Psychonaut/comments/2vbop2/psychedelics_effect_on_tourette_syndrome/
https://www.reddit.com/r/microdosing/comments/2cuz7u/what_are_the_effects_for_microdosing_mdma/
https://thethirdwave.co/microdosing-mdma/
https://www.quora.com/How-useful-is-microdosing-MDMA-for-socializing

https://www.nakedcapitalism.com/2013/12/tourettes-adventure-mind.html

Depression:
https://www.sciencealert.com/therapy-for-depression-gets-a-significant-boost-when-combined-with-psilocybin
https://thethirdwave.co/microdosing-depression/
https://www.reddit.com/r/microdosing/comments/6t8tdg/microdosing_mushrooms_for_depression/
https://theestablishment.co/the-magic-of-my-mushrooms-a-depressives-journey-to-microdosing-1675a7cf15a4
https://www.vice.com/en_us/article/8gk5wz/microdosing-psilocybin-depression-184
https://thethirdwave.co/psilocybin-end-life-treatment/

Alcoholism:
http://www.collective-evolution.com/2016/11/06/research-proves-psilocybins-ability-to-effectively-treat-alcoholism/
https://tonic.vice.com/en_us/article/7bx7bd/addicts-are-tripping-on-mushrooms-to-find-god-and-get-sober
https://www.zamnesia.com/blog-how-mushrooms-helped-me-quit-daily-and-abusive-drinking-n36
https://www.theguardian.com/society/2018/dec/04/alcohol-related-deaths-among-uk-women-highest-rate-10-years
https://www.ons.gov.uk/peoplepopulationandcommunity/healthandsocialcare/causesofdeath/bulletins/alcoholrelateddeathsintheunitedkingdom/previousReleases
https://www.ons.gov.uk/peoplepopulationandcommunity/healthandsocialcare/causesofdeath/datasets/alcoholrelateddeathsintheunitedkingdomreferencetable1
https://www.ons.gov.uk/peoplepopulationandcommunity/healthandsocialcare/causesofdeath/bulletins/alcoholrelateddeathsintheunitedkingdom/registeredin2017
https://www.drinkaware.co.uk/research/data/consequences/
https://alcoholchange.org.uk/alcohol-facts/fact-sheets/alcohol-statistics

https://www.who.int/substance_abuse/facts/alcohol/en/
https://www.statista.com/statistics/367890/alcohol-related-deaths-facts-worldwide/
https://medicalxpress.com/news/2018-09-excessive-million-people.html
https://civitas.org.uk/content/files/factsheet-alcoholcrime.pdf
http://www.ias.org.uk/uploads/pdf/factsheets/FS%20crime%20022017.pdf
http://www.ias.org.uk/Alcohol-knowledge-centre/Crime-and-social-impacts/Factsheets/Alcohol-related-crime-in-the-UK-what-do-we-know.aspx
https://www.addictioncenter.com/alcohol/alcohol-related-crime/
https://www.everydayhealth.com/womens-health/effects-of-alcohol-on-women.aspx
https://www.drinkaware.co.uk/alcohol-facts/health-effects-of-alcohol/alcohol-and-gender/alcohol-and-women/
https://www.niaaa.nih.gov/alcohol-health/special-populations-co-occurring-disorders/women
https://www.healthlinkbc.ca/health-topics/tk3598
https://www.poison.org/articles/2013-feb/alcohol-a-dangerous-poison-for-children
https://americanaddictioncenters.org/alcoholism-treatment/dangers-pregnancy
https://www.stanfordchildrens.org/en/topic/default?id=fetal-alcohol-syndrome-90-P02122
https://kidshealth.org/en/parents/fas.html
https://www.theguardian.com/society/2018/feb/11/parental-alcohol-abuse-linked-to-child-deaths-and-injuries
https://www.nhs.uk/conditions/sudden-infant-death-syndrome-sids/
http://www.ias.org.uk/Alcohol-knowledge-centre/Health-impacts/Factsheets/Alcohol-related-mortality-rates.aspx
https://www.who.int/violence_injury_prevention/publications/road_traffic/world_report/alcohol_en.pdf
https://www.ncbi.nlm.nih.gov/pubmed/24372493

https://www.who.int/news-room/fact-sheets/detail/road-traffic-injuries
https://assets.publishing.service.gov.uk/government/uploads/system/uploads/attachment_data/file/744077/reported-road-casualties-annual-report-2017.pdf
https://assets.publishing.service.gov.uk/government/uploads/system/uploads/attachment_data/file/732650/drink-drive-final-estimates-2016.pdf
https://digital.nhs.uk/data-and-information/publications/statistical/statistics-on-alcohol/2018/part-6
http://www.ias.org.uk/Alcohol-knowledge-centre/Drink-driving/Factsheets/Accidents-and-casualties.aspx
https://www.gov.uk/government/statistics/reported-road-casualties-in-great-britain-final-estimates-involving-illegal-alcohol-levels-2016
https://www.theguardian.com/society/2018/sep/26/uk-and-irish-teenagers-among-worst-in-europe-for-problem-drinking
https://www.drinkaware.co.uk/research/data/uk-underage-consumption/
https://www.drinkaware.co.uk/advice/underage-drinking/teenage-drinking/
https://news.sky.com/story/dramatic-decline-in-teenage-drinking-seen-across-the-uk-report-finds-11509092
https://www.familylives.org.uk/advice/teenagers/drugs-alcohol/underage-drinking/
https://www.nhs.uk/live-well/alcohol-support/
https://www.gov.uk/government/publications/alcohol-strategy

Prohibition
https://en.wikipedia.org/wiki/Prohibition_in_the_United_States
https://www.history.com/topics/roaring-twenties/prohibition
https://www.ncbi.nlm.nih.gov/pmc/articles/PMC1470475/

http://www.pbs.org/kenburns/prohibition/unintended-consequences/
https://www.alcoholproblemsandsolutions.org/effects-of-prohibition/

Smoking and Tobacco:
https://www.nhs.uk/common-health-questions/lifestyle/what-are-the-health-risks-of-smoking/
https://www.nhs.uk/smokefree/why-quit/smoking-health-problems
https://www.cancerresearchuk.org/health-professional/cancer-statistics/risk/tobacco
http://ash.org.uk/category/information-and-resources/fact-sheets/
http://ash.org.uk/information-and-resources/fact-sheets/the-economics-of-tobacco/
https://www.mentalhealth.org.uk/a-to-z/s/smoking-and-mental-health
https://digital.nhs.uk/data-and-information/publications/statistical/statistics-on-smoking/statistics-on-smoking-england-2018/content
https://www.verywellmind.com/global-smoking-statistics-for-2002-2824393
https://ourworldindata.org/smoking
http://www.euro.who.int/en/health-topics/disease-prevention/tobacco/data-and-statistics

Addiction:
https://www.gatewayfoundation.org/substance-abuse-treatment-programs/effects-of-drug-abuse/
https://www.mentalhelp.net/articles/signs-symptoms-effects-of-addiction/
https://www.altamirarecovery.com/drug-addiction/long-term-effects-drug-addiction/
https://www.altamirarecovery.com/drug-addiction/causes-effects-drug-addiction/

https://www.addictioncenter.com/addiction/addiction-in-the-uk/

Gateway to Drugs:
https://www.drugabuse.gov/publications/research-reports/marijuana/marijuana-gateway-drug
https://www.ncjrs.gov/App/Publications/abstract.aspx?ID=161247
https://americanaddictioncenters.org/the-real-gateway-drug
https://www.rivermendhealth.com/resources/alcohol-gateway-drug-cocaine/
https://www.drugwarfacts.org/chapter/drug_prison
https://www.theguardian.com/society/2018/oct/11/out-of-control-prison-watchdog-warns-of-synthetic-drug-crisis
https://www.acepnow.com/article/alcohol-tobacco-marijuana-true-gateway-drugs/

Mental Illness:
https://www.psychiatry.org/patients-families/what-is-mental-illness
http://www.businessinsider.de/psychedelics-depression-anxiety-alcoholism-mental-illness-2017-1?r=USandIR=T
https://www.huffingtonpost.com/entry/fundamental-psychedelic-drugs_us_5912109de4b050bdca60126c
https://www.rollingstone.com/culture/features/how-doctors-treat-mental-illness-with-psychedelic-drugs-w470673
http://www.howtousepsychedelics.org/
http://healthland.time.com/2012/12/07/magic-mushroom-drug-shows-promise-in-treating-addictions-and-cancer-anxiety/

PTSD:
https://www.nhs.uk/conditions/post-traumatic-stress-disorder-ptsd/
The differences between PTSD and C-PTSD:

https://www.talkspace.com/blog/2018/03/complex-ptsd-versus-standard-ptsd/
https://maps.org/news/multimedia-library/5321-using-psychedelic-drugs-to-treat-mental-disorders
https://maps.org/research/articles/6230-the-veteran-psychedelics-for-ptsd-what-a-long-strange-trip-it-s-been
https://www.militarytimes.com/news/your-army/2018/05/09/psychedelic-drug-provides-relief-for-veterans-with-ptsd/

OCD:
https://iocdf.org/about-ocd/
https://www.anxietybc.com/parenting/obsessive-compulsive-disorder
https://thethirdwave.co/psychedelics-ocd/
http://www.maps.org/research-archive/psilo/azproto.html
https://www.reddit.com/r/Drugs/comments/48ryiy/lsd_ocd/
https://www.maps.org/news-letters/v12n2/12217rs.html
https://www.reddit.com/r/OCD/comments/3si5dq/anybody_tried_microdosing_psilocybin_for_ocd/

Terminal illness:
https://www.mariecurie.org.uk/who/terminal-illness-definition
https://www.nhs.uk/conditions/end-of-life-care/coping-with-a-terminal-illness/
https://thethirdwave.co/psilocybin-end-life-treatment/
http://www.maps.org/news/multimedia-library/3012-how-psychedelic-drugs-can-help-patients-face-death
http://reset.me/story/psilocybin-helps-terminal-cancer-patients-find-new-ways-of-coping/
http://howtousepsychedelics.org/illness/
https://psychedelictimes.com/psilocybin-mushrooms/psilocybin-and-end-of-life-anxiety-reducing-stress-for-terminal-cancer-patients/

Chemotherapy:
https://www.cancer.net/survivorship/long-term-side-effects-cancer-treatment
https://www.nuffieldtrust.org.uk/resource/cancer-survival-rates
https://www.ncbi.nlm.nih.gov/pmc/articles/PMC2360753/
https://onlinelibrary.wiley.com/doi/full/10.3322/caac.21349
https://www.telegraph.co.uk/science/2016/08/30/chemotherapy-warning-as-hundreds-die-from-cancer-fighting-drugs/
https://www.collective-evolution.com/2018/05/04/new-study-reveals-many-cancer-patients-are-killed-by-chemotherapy-not-the-cancer/
https://www.gov.uk/government/news/new-findings-on-post-chemotherapy-deaths-using-world-first-phe-cancer-data
http://cancerres.aacrjournals.org/content/68/21/8643

Parkinson's:
https://parkinson.org/understanding-parkinsons/what-is-parkinsons
http://ourparkinsonsplace.blogspot.de/2017/10/magic-mushrooms-may-reset-brains-of.html
https://www.drugtimes.org/hallucinogens-culture/lsd-and-parkinsons-disease.html
https://www.reddit.com/r/Psychonaut/comments/5mi3v2/lsd_or_mdma_a_possible_treatmentrelief_for/

Multiple Sclerosis and Autoimmune:
https://www.nationalmssociety.org/What-is-MS/Definition-of-MS
https://www.reddit.com/r/Psychonaut/comments/5mi3v2/lsd_or_mdma_a_possible_treatmentrelief_for/
http://www.braintalkcommunities.org/showthread.php/101906-Psychedelics-and-MS
https://www.ncbi.nlm.nih.gov/pmc/articles/PMC4500993/

https://www.forbes.com/sites/emilywillingham/2015/08/04/why-did-my-grandmother-try-lsd-for-multiple-sclerosis-in-the-1960s/
https://www.reddit.com/r/microdosing/comments/8rqx81/any_other_microdosers_have_ms/
https://www.thisisms.com/forum/viewtopic.php?t=24133
https://www.ajmc.com/conferences/nei-2017/the-therapeutic-potential-of-marijuana-and-psychedelics

Micro-dosing and other Dosages:

https://thethirdwave.co/microdosing-mushrooms/
https://entheonation.com/blog/microdosing-magic-mushrooms-health-benefits-psilocybin-mushrooms-microdoses/
https://www.trufflemagic.com/blog/microdosing-magic-mushrooms/
https://www.reddit.com/r/mushrooms/comments/4os5ux/magic_mushroom_experience_based_on_different/
https://erowid.org/plants/mushrooms/mushrooms_dose.shtml

Mushroom Side-Effects:

https://thethirdwave.co/psychedelics/shrooms/
https://selfhacked.com/blog/psilocybin/
https://addictionresource.com/drugs/shrooms/effects-of-magic-mushrooms/

LSD:
https://thethirdwave.co/lsd-history/
http://www.psychedelic-library.org/hofmann.htm
https://thethirdwave.co/microdosing-with-lsd/
https://thethirdwave.co/volumetric-lsd/
https://www.reddit.com/r/Drugs/comments/1in13d/taking_lsd_for_first_time_need_you_to_review_my/

https://www.selfhacked.com/blog/experience-lsd/
https://drugs-forum.com/threads/lsd-experiences.9499/
https://www.verywellmind.com/what-does-it-feel-like-to-get-high-on-acid-21886
https://www.verywellmind.com/what-does-it-feel-like-to-get-high-on-acid-21886
https://www.reddit.com/r/Drugs/comments/34i8c7/1plsd_100µg_first_time_trip_report/
https://freedomandfulfilment.com/1p-lsd-experience-trip-report-50µg/
https://www.dmt-nexus.me/forum/default.aspx?g=postsandt=71704
https://www.reddit.com/r/Drugs/comments/3l6jjd/lsd_versus_1plsd/
https://erowid.org/experiences/exp.php?ID=106684
https://www.qualityhealth.com/health-lifestyle-articles/medical-uses-lsd
https://www.selfhacked.com/blog/lsd-lysergic-acid-diethylamide/
https://psy-minds.com/eleusinian-mysteries-ancient-greece/

Famous LSD and Psychedelics Users:
http://theconversation.com/lsd-microdosing-is-trending-in-silicon-valley-but-can-it-actually-make-you-more-creative-72747
https://www.huffingtonpost.com/entry/psychedelic-microdosing-research_us_569525afe4b09dbb4bac9db8
https://www.theatlantic.com/health/archive/2017/01/ayelet-lsd-microdosing/513035/
https://www.psychologytoday.com/us/blog/unique-everybody-else/201212/the-spirituality-psychedelic-drug-users
https://www.salon.com/2013/08/16/10_famous_geniuses_who_used_drugs_and_were_better_off_for_it_partner/
http://howtousepsychedelics.org/famous/
https://www.collective-evolution.com/2015/01/11/8-famous-people-whose-creativity-innovation-was-inspired-by-lsd/

MDMA:
https://thethirdwave.co/mdma/
https://www.huffingtonpost.com/2015/05/01/mdma-therapy_n_7181200.html
https://www.maps.org/news/media/6659-refinery29-the-couples-that-take-mdma-to-stay-together-2
https://www.inverse.com/article/27730-mdma-ecstasy-lsd-psychedelic-couples-therapy
https://www.yourtango.com/2016296859/why-using-mdma-couples-therapy-actually-saves-marriages
https://www.selfhacked.com/blog/mdma-2/

Micro-Dosing Experiences:
https://sites.google.com/view/microdosingpsychedelics/home
https://www.reddit.com/r/microdosing/comments/38sef1/7_months_microdosing_full_report_experiences_and/
https://thethirdwave.co/microdosing-experience/
http://www.jameswjesso.com/experiences-microdosing-psychedelics/
https://medium.com/@ericaavey/the-mental-and-metaphysical-effects-of-microdosing-lsd-72819896215d
https://www.theverge.com/2017/4/24/15403644/microdosing-lsd-acid-productivity-benefits-brain-studies
https://betterhumans.coach.me/how-one-year-of-microdosing-helped-my-career-relationships-and-happiness-715dbccdfae4
https://www.reddit.com/r/LSD/comments/4ib2y9/5_months_of_microdosing_report_and_long_term/
http://microdosing.info/long-term-effects-microdosing/

Headaches and Migraines:
https://psychedelictimes.com/2016/08/01/when-headaches-wont-stop-why-some-people-are-choosing-dmt-and-ayahuasca-to-treat-chronic-migraines/
https://www.gaia.com/article/psychedelics-for-migraines

https://migraineagain.com/get-ready-for-medicinal-mushrooms/
https://www.psymposia.com/magazine/psychedelic-survival/
https://howtousepsychedelics.org/cluster-headaches/
https://migrainemantras.com/2017/07/06/ocular-migraines-my-psychedelic-experience/
https://psychedelictimes.com/ayahuasca/when-headaches-wont-stop-why-some-people-are-choosing-dmt-and-ayahuasca-to-treat-chronic-migraines/

Schizophrenia:
https://www.bbrfoundation.org/what-is-schizophrenia-signs-symptoms-treatments
https://www.reddit.com/r/microdosing/comments/6ykz0k/family_history_of_schizophrenia/
https://thethirdwave.co/demonizing-psychedelics-schizophrenia/
https://www.mushroomery.org/forums/showflat.php/Number/14830527
http://www.news.com.au/national/lsd-reveals-schizophrenia-treatment/news-story/8779d8d22884c2a1ab7cc2dc85e89162
http://www.bluelight.org/vb/threads/823889-Psychedelics-and-schizophrenia
https://www.sciencedaily.com/releases/2015/12/151217111711.htm
https://www.sciencedaily.com/releases/2015/12/151217111711.htm
https://www.psychologytoday.com/us/blog/diagnosis-diet/201706/ketogenic-diets-psychiatric-disorders-new-2017-review
http://advancednutrition.me/ketogenic-diet-treats-schizophrenia-aids-bipolar-depression-and-weight-loss-say-scientists

Ayahuasca:
https://www.soul-herbs.com/ayahuasca-benefits/

http://www.medicinehunter.com/ayahuasca
https://www.warrior.do/ayahuasca/
https://www.reddit.com/r/Ayahuasca/comments/4lc8ru/how_did_your_life_change_after_ayahuasca/
https://www.selfhacked.com/blog/ayahuasca/

MAPS research group:
http://www.maps.org
https://www.maps.org/resources/students/181-so-you-want-to-be-a-psychedelic-researcher

Jesus, cannabis and Religion:
https://patients4medicalmarijuana.wordpress.com/2009/12/22/jesus-healed-using-Cannabis-study-shows/
https://en.wikipedia.org/wiki/Cannabis_and_religion
https://herb.co/marijuana/news/jesus-medical-marijuana-Cannabis
https://www.ranker.com/list/evidence-that-jesus-used-Cannabis/green-rush-daily
https://www.huffingtonpost.com/entry/psychedelic-drugs-religious-leaders_us_58750c36e4b02b5f858b350a

Spiritualism:
https://www.psychologytoday.com/blog/unique-everybody-else/201212/the-spirituality-psychedelic-drug-users
https://thethirdwave.co/psychedelics-spiritual/
https://www.maps.org/participate/participate-in-research/133-auxiliary-studies-not-sponsored-by-maps/2448-psychedelic-drugs-and-mystical-experiences
http://www.psychedelic-library.org/relmenu.htm
https://www.theguardian.com/science/2017/jul/08/religious-leaders-get-high-on-magic-mushrooms-ingredient-for-science

Cannabis:
History of cannabis:

https://en.wikipedia.org/wiki/Legal_history_of_Cannabis_in_the_United_States
http://www.idmu.co.uk/historical.htm

Benefits of cannabis:
https://azmarijuana.com/dans-stash/medicinal-benefits-marijuana-graph/
https://www.health.harvard.edu/blog/medical-marijuana-2018011513085
https://www.learngreenflower.com/articles/66/50-life-enhancing-benefits-of-Cannabis
www.learngreenflower.com/articles/574/medical-uses-of-Cannabis
http://www.encod.org/info/700-MEDICINAL-USES-OF-CANNABIS.html

Risks from cannabis:
https://www.nhs.uk/live-well/healthy-body/cannabis-the-facts/
https://www.drugabuse.gov/publications/drugfacts/marijuana
https://www.canada.ca/en/health-canada/services/drugs-medication/cannabis/health-effects/effects.html

Cannabis and Cancer Treatment:

https://www.healthline.com/health/rick-simpson-oil-cancer#research
https://medium.com/@ericgeisterfer/23-people-who-beat-cancer-using-cannabis-oil-only-c1b285e31d62
https://www.thestreet.com/lifestyle/health/rick-simpson-oil-14760699
http://www.pbso.ca/is-rick-simpson-oil-capable-of-treating-cancer/
https://www.cancer.org/treatment/treatments-and-side-effects/complementary-and-alternative-medicine/marijuana-and-cancer.html
https://www.projectcbd.org/medicine/cbd-thc-and-cancer

https://www.worldwidecancerresearch.org/who-we-are/cannabis/
http://www.cancer.ca/en/cancer-information/diagnosis-and-treatment/complementary-therapies/medical-cannabis-and-cannabinoids/?region=qc
https://integrativeonc.org/news/research-blog/277-does-cannabis-cure-cancer

Deaths from cannabis:
http://www.weedist.com/2012/06/marijuana-safer-than-peanuts/
https://www.sciencealert.com/physicians-refute-us-child-death-marijuana-link
https://www.promises.com/resources/overdose/many-people-died-weed/

Deaths from psychedelics:
https://infogram.com/annual-us-deaths-from-psychedelics-compared-to-other-causes-1gvew2ve5v5nmnj
https://www.ncbi.nlm.nih.gov/pmc/articles/PMC5867510/
https://www.ons.gov.uk/peoplepopulationandcommunity/birthsdeathsandmarriages/deaths/adhocs/005757numberofdeathsfromselectedpsychedelicsubstances1993to2014
https://deserthopetreatment.com/psychedelic-mushrooms/can-you-die/
https://www.iflscience.com/health-and-medicine/only-a-handful-of-people-in-history-have-ever-overdosed-on-lsd-this-is-what-happened-to-them/
https://www.theguardian.com/society/2017/may/23/study-hallucinogenic-mushrooms-safest-recreational-drug-lsd

Toxicology and related info:
http://whs.rocklinusd.org/documents/Science/Lethal_Dose_Table.pdf
https://www.brainprotips.com/adderall-overdose/
https://www.ncbi.nlm.nih.gov/pubmed/16086703

http://www.telegraph.co.uk/news/2017/06/13/daily-aspirin-behind-3000-deaths-year-study-suggests/
http://www.adjusthealth.info/usefull-info/news/25-40-000-deaths-in-usa-caused-by-aspirin-and-painkillers-every-year
https://drugfreeva.org/death-chart/
https://drugfree.org/learn/drug-and-alcohol-news/prescription-drugs-including-opioids-responsible-for-most-overdose-deaths/
https://www.drugfreeworld.ie/drugfacts/prescription/abuse-international-statistics.html
https://www.cdc.gov/drugoverdose/data/prescribing.html
https://www.cdc.gov/drugoverdose/data/otherdrugs.html
https://www.kff.org/other/state-indicator/opioid-overdose-deaths-by-type-of-opioid/
https://www.ncbi.nlm.nih.gov/pubmed/17536879
https://www.bbc.com/news/uk-45083167
http://www.eurad.net/en/research/new_research/Annual+figures+on+drug-related+deaths+in+UK.9UFRzK58.ips
https://www.independent.co.uk/news/uk/home-news/drug-deaths-record-high-statistics-opioids-fentanyl-carfentanyl-cocaine-spice-ons-laws-reform-a8479431.html

Botox:
https://www.ncbi.nlm.nih.gov/pmc/articles/PMC2840902/

Effects of Psilocybin:
http://www.psypost.org/2010/01/psychological-and-physiological-effects-of-psilocybin-48
https://www.mushroomery.org/forums/showflat.php/Number/20236315
https://www.ncbi.nlm.nih.gov/pubmed/14615876
http://www.bluelight.org/vb/threads/723357-psychedelics-and-hypertension-harm-reduction-please

Theresa May's Banning of Psychedelics:

https://www.theguardian.com/science/2015/dec/13/vaughan-bell-legal-highs-psychoactive-drugs-bill

Research Programmes and Reviews Regarding Research:
https://www.maps.org/resources/students/181-so-you-want-to-be-a-psychedelic-researcher
https://heffter.org/
https://www.nytimes.com/2017/07/17/upshot/can-psychedelics-be-therapy-allow-research-to-find-out.html
http://beckleyfoundation.org/
https://www.vox.com/2016/6/27/11544250/psychedelic-drugs-lsd-psilocybin-effects
https://www.frontiersin.org/research-topics/5512/psychedelic-drug-research-in-the-2first-century
http://reset.me/story/how-to-get-involved-in-the-psychedelic-renaissance/
https://motherboard.vice.com/en_us/article/pazeab/james-fadiman-lsd-microdosing-research
https://sites.google.com/view/microdosingpsychedelics/home

Fentanyl and Opioid Deaths:
https://www.theguardian.com/us-news/2017/dec/27/its-all-fentanyl-opioid-crisis-takes-shape-in-philadelphia-as-overdoses-surge
https://www.telegraph.co.uk/news/2018/01/31/deadly-fentanyl-behind-dramatic-doubling-synthetic-opioid-death/

Lists the Fentanyl Dosage for Kids:
https://online.epocrates.com/drugs/169102/fentanyl/Peds-Dosing

Victoria Aitkin and Paul Kenward:
https://www.clear-uk.org/victoria-atkins-mp-the-uk-drugs-minister-opposes-drugs-regulation-while-her-husband-grows-45-acres-of-Cannabis-under-government-licence/

https://www.independent.co.uk/news/uk/politics/drugs-minister-victoria-atkins-hypocrisy-Cannabis-paul-kenward-british-sugar-a8356056.html

William Hague:
https://www.bbc.com/news/uk-politics-44526156

How the Brain Works:
https://waitbutwhy.com/2017/04/neuralink.html#part2

Serotonin:
https://sapiensoup.com/serotonin

How Psychedelics Affect the Brain:
https://sapiensoup.com/brain-on-psychedelic-drugs

Mormon Church and Stance Against cannabis:
https://herb.co/marijuana/news/mormon-churchs-Cannabis-illegal-utah
https://www.civilized.life/articles/mormon-church-big-Pharma-stocks/

NHS Potential Savings from Legalising cannabis:
https://iea.org.uk/publications/joint-venture/

Psychopathy, Sociopathy and Narcissism:
James Fallon *The Psychopath Inside*
Andy McNab and Kevin Dutton *The Good Psychopath's Guide*
Paul Babaik and Robert D Hare *Snakes in Suits*
Kevin Dutton *The Wisdom of Psychopaths*
Martha Stout *The Sociopath Next Door*
Craig Malkin *Rethinking Narcissism*

Psychopath, Sociopath and Narcissist Tests:

These are the two tests I used to determine my psychopathy, sociopathy and narcissistic respectively.

Psychopath:
https://www.healthyplace.com/psychological-tests/psychopath-test.-am-i-a-psychopath

Sociopath:
https://www.healthyplace.com/psychological-tests/sociopath-test-am-i-a-sociopath

Narcissist:
https://openpsychometrics.org/tests/NPI/

Differences Between a Psychopath, Sociopath and Narcissist:
https://theydiffer.com/difference-between-psychopath-sociopath-and-narcissist/
https://www.psychologytoday.com/intl/blog/wicked-deeds/201401/how-tell-sociopath-psychopath

What is Anti-Social Personality Disorder:
https://www.psychologytoday.com/us/conditions/antisocial-personality-disorder

An Anti-social Personality Disorder test:
https://www.psycom.net/antisocial-personality-disorder-sociopath-test/

Users of Psychedelics:
https://www.hallucinogens.org/lsd/francis-crick.html
https://www.salon.com/2013/08/16/10_famous_geniuses_who_used_drugs_and_were_better_off_for_it_partner/
http://howtousepsychedelics.org/famous/
https://www.ranker.com/list/celebrities-who-owe-their-careers-to-psychedelics/jacob-shelton

Ricaute's MDMA Report:
http://www.maps.org/research-archive/mdma/studyresponse.html

https://en.wikipedia.org/wiki/Retracted_article_on_dopaminergic_neurotoxicity_of_MDMA
http://science.sciencemag.org/content/301/5639/1479.2

Other Quotes:
Psychologytoday.com
https://thethirdwave.co/psychedelic-quotes/
https://en.wikiquote.org/wiki/Talk:Paul_McCartney
http://quotes.liberty-tree.ca/quotes/drugs
Vincent Thnay: Quotes Worthy
https://www.azquotes.com/quote/580102
https://www.goodreads.com/author/quotes/1201.Daniel_Pinchbeck
C. G. Leukefeld, et al.: Drug Use: A Reference Handbook
Clay S. Conrad: Jury Nullification: The Evolution of a Doctrine
http://volokh.com/2013/01/05/gary-becker-and-kevin-murphy-on-the-failure-of-the-war-on-drugs/
https://www.quora.com/Did-Steve-Jobs-claim-that-taking-LSD-was-a-profound-experience-one-of-the-most-important-things-in-his-life
https://creation.com/dry-land-green-grass-juicy-fruit-day-3
https://www.azquotes.com/quote/558034
https://www.goodreads.com/quotes/
http://www.choicesunlimited.ca/famous-medical-quotes/
T.S. Eliot: The Four Quartets
https://www.azquotes.com/quotes/topics/shame-and-guilt.html
Buddha: The Kalama Sutta
https://www.poetryfoundation.org/poems/44272/the-road-not-taken

www.ingramcontent.com/pod-product-compliance
Lightning Source LLC
Chambersburg PA
CBHW070459120526
44590CB00013B/692